AIDS

AIDS

INTERVENING WITH HIDDEN GRIEVERS

Barbara O. Dane

AND

Samuel O. Miller

Foreword by
GEORGE GETZEL

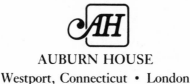

AUBURN HOUSE
Westport, Connecticut • London

155.91
DI7a

Library of Congress Cataloging-in-Publication Data

Dane, Barbara O.
    AIDS : intervening with hidden grievers / Barbara O. Dane and
Samuel O. Miller ; foreword by George Getzel.
        p. cm.
    Includes bibliographical references and index.
    ISBN 0–86569–028–6 (alk. paper)
    1. Bereavement—Psychological aspects.   2. AIDS (Disease)—
Psychological aspects.   3. AIDS (Disease)—Patients—Family
relationships.   4. Grief therapy.   I. Miller, Samuel   O.   II. Title.
    [DNLM: 1. Acquired Immunodeficiency Syndrome—psychology.
2. Bereavement.   3. Social Support.   WD 208 D179a]
RC455.4.L67D36   1992
362.1'969792—dc20   92–10959
DNLM/DLC
for Library of Congress

British Library Cataloguing in Publication Data is available.

Library of Congress Catalog Card Number: 92–10959
ISBN: 0–86569–028–6

First published in 1992

Auburn House, 88 Post Road West, Westport, CT 06881
An imprint of Greenwood Publishing Group, Inc.

Printed in the United States of America

The paper used in this book complies with the
Permanent Paper Standard issued by the National
Information Standards Organization (Z39.48–1984).

10 9 8 7 6 5 4 3 2 1

Contents

Foreword

Ten years have past since the recognition of AIDS began, and now the disease is an integral part of the broad culture and everyday life. More than two hundred thousand Americans have been diagnosed with the disease and more than a million persons are infected with the Human Immune Deficiency Virus (HIV) associated with the prospective occurrence of serious illness years later. AIDS and HIV have become emblematic of Death as we approach the closing of the next millennium.

Justifiably to date, major attention has been given to the prevention of HIV transmission and the care of the sick and the dying. Recently, more attention have been given to the role of caregivers: the kin and friends of people with AIDS who undergo a series of crises that may have pernicious social and emotional consequences. Typically, such discussions of caregivers do not adequately address the reality that the problem of AIDS persists after a PWA dies, at a significant if not at a traumatic level, for grieving and bereaved loved ones.

Sadly the denial of grief goes hand-in-glove with the denial of death. For this reason alone, we should celebrate the wise analysis of Barabara Dane and Sam Miller, even if we may be discomforted by their subject matter. I humbly recommend that readers find the courage to proceed in the exploration of bereavement and AIDS as the authors suggest. In the second decade we will have to come to terms with the heavy toll of death that lives in the souls of millions of survivors of the AIDS pandemic in this country and throughout the world.

The depth of the AIDS trauma for survivors can only be understood in the context of the hurt and the remembrance of any group of people who suffers mass bereavement that has stark political and cultural meanings. Perhaps, the analogies of war and genocide in the twentieth century are apt ones to understand the long term implications of the ongoing AIDS death toll. For example, it took in the cases of survivors of the Nazis genocide and Turkish massacre of Armenians several decades to be accepted by the world in terms of the profound dimension of unabating grief.

As a personally bereaved survivor, I find the World Health Organization's prediction of 40 million cases of AIDS and 10 million surviving children on this planet in the next ten years a very real prospect. In my beloved New York City, we anticipated whole families desolated and 20,000 AIDS orphans.

As we pause aghast and in silence, let this book serve as a "wake-up call" to activate humane concern and action.

George S. Getzel, DSW
Professor, Hunter College
New York City

Acknowledgments

Many have contributed to the thinking that led us to write this volume. We owe our greatest debt to family, friends, colleagues, persons with AIDS and their bereaved survivors who have inspired and encouraged us with their tireless effort, good humor, shared grief and hope to help us think logically, write coherently and be empatically attuned. We are deeply grateful to our colleagues who have contributed their precious time, support and case materials to assemble this project.

Among those to whom we are especially indebted are Sidney Paul Dane and significant others, for providing on-going support and confidence in our abilities to collaborate this venture, to maintain our sanity, and to articulate our values and understanding of what it is like to be a survivor grieving the death of a loved one from AIDS.

We also want to thank Franciska Caldwell, our former student whose extensive research provided numerous articles which supported writing this book, and Dr. George Getzel for his contributions. Finally, we want to thank our colleagues from New York University and Columbia Universaty Schools of Social Work for providing us with support, stimulation and encouragement. We also want to thank our students, clients and field instructs, whose exchange of theoretical ideas, practice wisdom, questions, uncertainties and desire for understanding provided the force to conceptualize our ideas more carefully and to put them into communicable form.

Finally we also thank John Harney, Editorial Director of Auburn House, for his unintrusive support and good advice.

AIDS

Introduction

As the epidemic of the acquired immune deficiency syndrome (AIDS) enters a second decade, the number of survivors, families and loved ones of people who have died from the disease, continues to increase. Walker (1987) has documented that each family system has, on average, seven to ten survivors. These figures do not include neighbors, friends, co-workers or others outside the family system. Death is a unique and personal experience. There is no way to predict how a person will respond to loss. There are, however, common and universal feelings that help the bereaved feel connected to others who have had a similar experience. In this book, we discuss what families, lovers, friends and professionals have told us about how they were affected by the death of a person from AIDS, giving us an understanding of their experiences, their reactions and how they coped with and resolved their grief.

Despite the statistics we have available about the number of persons who have died from or who are currently diagnosed with and likely to die from AIDS, there has been little available information on the number of grievers left behind and how they have coped when a loved one has died from AIDS. For more than a decade, this population of bereaved survivors has been overlooked in our psychological literature and, to a lesser extent, by the professional community.

The question of whether or when to treat the bereaved has always been controversial. Freud (1917) asserted that the normal processes of grieving should not be interfered with, and there is a widespread belief that "time alone heals." Studies unrelated to AIDS, but concerned with bereavement (Schoenberg, et al. 1974; Parkes 1975) show that the time taken for healing is much longer than formerly thought, and note that a vast number of survivors are highly vulnerable to physical and mental deterioration. These facts lead to questions regarding the potential for primary and secondary intervention.

The perils of survivorship have led to a growing appreciation of the grief and mourning process. Bettelheim (1979), writing about surviving the Nazi holocaust, offers a framework for understanding survivorship: "survivorship consists of two closely related, but separate issues. First is the original trauma. . . . Second, there are the life-long aftereffects of such a trauma, which seem to require very special forms of mastery if one is not to succumb to them (24-25).

This framework can be applied to survivors of airline crashes, fires, earthquakes, tornadoes, floods, mass kidnappings, war-related events and AIDS. The stressful emotions that survivors experience are powerful and touch off unconscious psychological reactions that jeopardize their lives.

In general, the psychosocial aspects of survivorship of a sudden or prolonged death are similar to those experienced by AIDS survivors, although we are far less knowledgeable about the impact of death as applied specifically to AIDS survivors. What makes AIDS survivors distinct is that AIDS is related to cultural taboos concerning homosexuality, sex and drugs that stigmatize individuals in their adaptation and response to the grieving process.

This book is intended to fill a glaring gap in our knowledge of survivors grieving the death of a person with AIDS. While we cannot hope to have uncovered the full meaning of this event, there is much that we have discovered that sheds light on it. We discuss how loved ones, family, friends and significant others are likely to respond when death from AIDS occurs. We also show how survivors are able to find their way through the fears and stigma often associated with AIDS, and how they transcend their losses.

The reader will find an interweaving of themes, ideas, feelings and experiences from one chapter to another.

In Chapter 1, we present a brief overview of theories on grief and bereavement, not necessarily unique to survivors of people with AIDS (PWAs). The theories lend a perspective on how survivors grieve and cope with the death of a loved one.

Chapter 2 presents information about the AIDS crisis and on additional social issues with which survivors have to deal in resolving their grief.

Chapter 3 discusses the unique aspects and major concerns in being an AIDS survivor coping with the death of a loved one.

Chapters 4 through 8 are practice-related. Personal and clinical experiences of survivors are interwoven with existing theory and research. Attention is focused on several specific subgroups of survivors: children and adolescents (Chapter 4); mothers and female partners, lovers and friends (Chapter 5); gay lovers and friends (Chapter 6); families of homosexual and bisexual men (Chapter 7); and inner-city families (Chapter 8).

The grief of practitioners is discussed in Chapter 9, and we offer strategies for coping with their bereavement.

The contents of this book are drawn from our clinical experience with survivors, from interviews with survivors of deceased PWAs, and from on-going groups and workshops and teaching seminars for professionals and students working with persons with AIDS and their survivors. Although interviewing the bereaved is a delicate process, and sometimes can feel intrusive, those approached were pleased to be part of this undertaking. Professionals have generously contributed their time and knowledge gained from their practice to describe their emotionally draining but uplifting work with persons with AIDS and their bereaved survivors.

The book is written primarily for mental health professionals who are called upon to render services in the aftermath of a loved one's death from AIDS. The major aims of this book are: (1) to present a state-of-the-art review of existing information about survivorship and bereavement, and to increase the reader's knowledge of the problem of AIDS survivors; (2) to provide firsthand information about clinical issues encountered by AIDS survivors in a variety of clinical settings; and (3) to increase mental health professionals' awareness of the need to develop models that can be tried and evaluated for their effectiveness in treating survivors of AIDS.

This book should help mental health practitioners appreciate how survivors of people who died from AIDS can be helped, their grief understood, their sense of self reinforced and their establishment of new relationships encouraged. It is usually difficult to read and work with grief and bereavement without looking inward. Consequently, the reader's own feelings of attachment and loss will be quietly encountered and revisited. It is our hope that this material will help develop a more sensitive, humanistic understanding of what the death of a loved one from AIDS means in our modern society.

CHAPTER 1

Overview of Theories on Grief and Bereavement

AIDS is a harsh teacher, imposing on us a painful tutorial in grief and mourning that has returned death to the vocabulary of everyday life. An abiding legacy of the AIDS epidemic will be its effect on survivors. As the epidemic calls into question the mortality of civilization, we are forced to acknowledge our ideal of health, and the tensions of harmonizing in the midst of society's differences. One thing we now have in common, despite early efforts to confine AIDS to a distinctive group of others, is the strong sense that the infection, death, grief and mourning touch us all.

The public's current image of persons with AIDS is no longer only of those who died after anonymous encounters in bathhouses or repeated trips to shoot-up galleries. The bravery of Magic Johnson, Ryan White and Kimberly Bergalis provides a moving symbol of the losses sustained from the disease. A huge national quilt of a thousand squares is a flowing monument not to painful death but to personal memories of a community of survivors. There is now a compelling voice that sends the message that grieving a death from AIDS is both a private and public affair.

Dying from AIDS is usually quite protracted. There may be many years from initial HIV infection to the development of clinical symptoms; days to years between the development of symptoms and the development of diagnosed AIDS; and perhaps another year or several years until death. This lengthy time between the AIDS diagnosis and death leads to many differences in how survivors respond to the grief process. It would be erroneous to generalize that all people surviving death from a loved one to AIDS will conform to the process as defined by the models of grief discussed in this chapter.

In many ways each survivor has a unique relationship with the deceased and will experience the death and grief differently. Yet, each experience is also similar to the experiences of others in many respects. If we can come to understand the commonalities of bereavement that underlie loss, as out-lined in this chapter, we may come to know better the great variability that survivors face when they cope with the death of a loved one from AIDS. Understanding these nuances will enhance the professional's response to this bereaved population. Further, it can predict some of the professional's dif-ficulties, and can move clinicians to seek help for themselves when their own coping abilities become overburdened.

OVERVIEW

Contemporary models of grief are largely based on the attachment behavior of young primates or young humans observed when separated from their mothers (Bowlby 1969, 1973, 1980b; Parkes 1972; Raphael 1983; Worden 1982). A less prominent but often-quoted theoretical approach derives from the psychoanalytic literature (Volkan 1981), which bases its model of grief on the internalization of the lost object. When we examine the grief of loved ones after the death of a person to AIDS, neither the attachment model nor the psychoanalytic model seems to account adequately for many of the phe-nomena observed, although we use these models as a frame of reference. Grief, as we define it here, is a state of physical and mental unease, caused by the realization that a significant person or part of the self is lost. The response to this loss is reflected in how the person feels, behaves and thinks. The complex grief that survivors experience after the death of a loved one to AIDS is both a continuation of the complex dynamics by which the attachment to the deceased was developed, and a response to the stigma of AIDS in the environment.

It may be impossible to define a typical bereavement reaction, since there are so many variables that contribute to the form and length of bereavement, as well as to the feelings of the bereaved. There is no way to predict how a loved one will respond, since each death will be experienced differently by each person. Each suffers grief in her or his own personal way and within her or his own time frame.

Death threatens us with the abrogation of ourselves and all that we love and value. Each of us is continuously subject to the threat of death, and our experiences in life often involve a loss of some kind, whether physical or symbolic. All of us are grievers, and themes of loss confront us over the life span.

The practitioner's challenge in responding to loss is to understand the unique aspects of the survivor's grief and mourning process. An assessment is based on how the person died, the nature and closeness of the relationship to the deceased, the stages of bereavement, prior death experiences and varying physical and emotional needs, as well as religious, cultural and ethnic differences.

This chapter presents in a general manner certain behavior patterns and attitudes that dominate the response patterns of some survivors at various points during their bereavement. Helping an individual and family rebuild their lives after the death of a loved one is a significant task for mental health professionals. This task is complicated in AIDS bereavement by a number of special issues in addition to those raised by the grieving related to any loss.

THEORETICAL UNDERPINNINGS OF GRIEF AND BEREAVEMENT

To understand better how survivors react to loss and to help them reshape their lives in a more positive way, it is essential first to reexamine some of the most impressive systematic studies and theories in the field of bereavement.

Lindemann (1944) was the first contemporary major theorist to contribute to the understanding of survivor problems. He points out that it would be more reasonable to help the survivor appreciate that the pain of grief is a normal reaction to the stress caused by the loss. Elisabeth Kübler-Ross's (1969) work, *On Death and Dying*, has helped professionals open up these areas for further exploration.

Kohut's (1971) theory of the self offers a conceptualization, within a normative development context, which may provide further insight into the experience of loss. He proposes that the infant, with a cohesive yet archaic sense of self, requires an environment in which it feels complemented in order to survive. The adult provides this complementarity by becoming a selfobject for the child, and the child experiences this merger with the self-object as providing a sense of cohesion and wholeness. The selfobject, by responding with approval to the child's grandiose fantasies, acts as a tension regulator, thereby relieving feelings of helplessness in the child. The functions provided by the selfobject are gradually internalized, and the child develops a capacity to tolerate victory and defeat as well as acceptance and rejection. Kohut further points out that the need for selfobjects continues throughout adult life and that they are required for psychological survival. In the grief process the experience of the loss of the object, unless resolved, is disruptive to survival.

Palumbo (1981), in discussing the loss of a love object through death, describes the process as characterized by initial shock, disbelief (especially if the death is unexpected) and denial. Eventually the defense of denial gives way to a gradual acceptance of reality; the painful feelings associated with the anticipation of lost attachment are expressed through the grieving process.

The natural response to loss is grief. The struggle to accommodate loss is a fact of life that permeates each stage of human development. It typifies much of the individual's efforts to come to terms with the issue of mortality (Martin 1989). Grief has often been described as an illness from which the mourner eventually recovers (Parkes 1972). If grief is indeed an illness, the mourner must assume that something is wrong with her/himself, feeling assailed by intense and unfamiliar emotions following the loss and believing also in a "cure" from the pain and disruption in finding the right treatment.

Engel (1961) describes grief as a deep, painful psychological wound similar to the trauma one sustains in a severe physical injury. Grief work, the resolving of the relationship, is analogous to a scab laid down to nurture and close the wound. Since grief work is so painful, survivors may suppress their emotions in an effort to stop the pain. If one chooses to avoid the painful experience, withdrawing from the pain and trying to go on with life without dealing with the wound, there may be sharp, unrelated angry outbursts, painful relationships, irritable behaviors, depression and other symptomatic behaviors (Redmond 1989).

Hoagland (1984) points out that one of the most important discoveries about bereavement is that the symptoms tend to follow a predictable course over time. One must go through grief work, grieving for one's loss (or sometimes multiple losses, as in AIDS deaths) in order to heal the wound. When the wound is healed there will be a scar, but it will be a healed psychological wound.

Bowlby's (1977) attachment theory provides a framework for us to conceptualize the need in humans to make strong, affectionate emotional bonds with one another. The theory also helps us understand the depth of the reaction when the attachment is threatened (severe illness) or broken (death). People develop attachments early in life to meet the need for security and safety. The attachments are directed to a few individuals, and endure throughout most of one's lifetime. Bowlby regards attachment behavior as distinct from the biological needs for food or sexual behavior. When the bond is threatened, the normal biological reaction is to protest, seek, and restore the attachment. Searching and seeking behaviors ensue. Infants who fail to thrive because their needs for bonding and trusting another have gone unmet exhibit this reaction.

Worden (1982) notes that if these infant needs are not satisfied, apathy, withdrawal and despair are evident. Later in life, the difficulty may manifest itself in failure to establish trust with another human being and in angry acting-out behaviors. The failure-to-thrive infant is grieving for the loss of an emotional attachment and cannot trust that others will provide safety and security.

The crisis of loss is experienced by each of us throughout our lives. We search to restore, replace and adapt to change by severing our attachment to persons we may lose or have lost. Each loss results in the need to do grief work (Lindemann and Green 1953), which requires the expenditure of both physical and emotional energy.

Caplan (1961) states that if one is to survive the losses suffered in a tragic crisis, one must hold up the image of what was, reviewing in detail, reviving memories of what life once had been. Only then, can one begin to accept the challenge and begin the process of resolution.

THE DIMENSIONS OF NORMAL BEREAVEMENT

The sensitive professional who encounters a bereaved person is immediately aware that this person needs help, but the nature of the help that is needed is often unclear. Grief is easy to detect clinically, but whether grief is unresolved and pathological is difficult to define operationally. Just asking the survivor how she/he feels about the deceased usually prompts the reactions of grief. The clinician who works with a bereaved person must understand the many dimensions of grief and respond to individual survivors based on their unique rhythms.

Freud (1917) in his classic paper "Mourning and Melancholia" undertakes to define the normal process of grief. He asserts that grief is prompted by loss and that this loss need not only involve a death; he notes that grief is a normal and expected process, and implies a self-healing aspect to grief that, under normal conditions, will occur without intervention. Anna Freud (1957) defines mourning as

the reaction to the loss of a loved person, or to the loss of some abstraction which has taken the place of one, such as one's country, liberty, an ideal, and so on. . . . It is also well worth notice that, although mourning involves grave departures from the normal attitude to life, it never occurs to us to regard it as a pathological condition and to refer it to medical treatment. We rely on its being overcome after a certain lapse of time, and we look upon any interference with it as useless or even harmful. (243-44).

Sigmund Freud's grave departures from the normal process of mourning is described in the following characteristics associated with grief: a profound painful dejection; cessation of interest in the outside world; loss of capacity to love; inhibition of activity by withdrawal from any activity not connected with thoughts of the lost person.

Unlike Freud, Bowlby's (1960) break with traditional psychoanalytic views of loss includes rejection of the abstract concepts of psychic energy and drive. He forges a link with research in cognitive psychology and human information processing in developing his theory of attachment and loss. Attachment is a dynamic, instinctive, goal-directed behavior.

For Bowlby, loss and mourning, which can be applied to the grief process, result from temporary or permanent separation from attachment figures. Two key elements of the mourning process involve withdrawal of emotional investment and preparations for investing in a new relationship.

The major distinction between Bowlby's theory and those of Freud and his followers lies in how these elements are achieved and how affectional bonds are conceptualized. Freud (1917) sees identification as the origin of emotional ties with an object, while for Bowlby (1980), attachment is responsible for the development of affectional bonds. In addition, traditional psychoanalysis views the function of grief as a means of detaching from the individual who is gone. Bowlby's theory implies that, far from promoting separation, grief has the biological function of promoting reunion between the survivor and the deceased person. Only in the case of permanent loss do the most obvious features of grief extinguish with no reunion occurring.

STAGES OF GRIEF

The notion that the grieving process takes place in a series of stages, similar to Kübler-Ross's (1969) psychological stages in the dying process, has been developed by a number of writers (Gorer 1967; Glick, Weiss & Parkes 1974; Parkes 1972; Bowlby 1960; Kavanaugh 1974; Schneider 1984). Different theorists suggest there are three, four, five or even eight stages in the grief process.

The first stage in almost all formulations is described as a period of shock, numbness or disbelief, lasting a few days or at most a few weeks. Loss of self-control, reduced energy, lack of motivation, bewilderment, disorientation and a loss of perspective characterize this initial period in the grieving process.

Following the first stage, the remaining two to eight stages entail a long period of grief and related emotions (pining, depression, guilt, anger), in which the individual tries to find some meaning to the loss. A failure to resolve any stage may mean a blocking of the grief, which in turn may lead to a pathological outcome or may mean residuals of the loss could influence the later life course of the bereaved.

In a large percentage of cases, the bereavement process runs its course after approximately a year or more following the death. By that time, the bereaved individual has given up any hope of recovering the deceased and is ready to reorganize her/his life and focus on new objects of interest.

As with any theory of developmental stages or periods, there is a danger that the stages of grief theory will be interpreted as a fixed sequence through which all bereaved people must pass. Bugen (1977) has cautioned about possible misinterpretations of stage theories. He notes that the different stages of grief blend together and overlap, are not necessarily successive, vary in intensity and duration and are not experienced by every bereaved person.

Consequently, he argues that the stage theories are only descriptive accounts of various emotional stages experienced by bereaved persons. We would add that a particular mourner may not go through all the stages, and not necessarily in a specific order.

Research evidence supporting the concept of stages of grief is neither extensive nor convincing. Robert Fulton (1987) takes issue with the Freudian influence in our understanding of the process of mourning—namely, that the process is "time-bounded," lasting a year or two, and that the essential task of grieving is to give up one's attachment to the deceased ("decathexis"). Fulton's research on widows indicates that for many, if not for most widows, the work of mourning does not end. In addition, mothers of stillborn children and women who have had miscarriages have grief reactions that do not fit the attachment theories. Like an amputation or dismemberment, the loss continues.

CHRONIC SORROW

The concept of shadow grief was first revealed in the book *Motherhood and Mourning: Perinatal Death* (Peppers & Knapp 1980). These authors found the lingering effects of grief to be quite prominent among mothers who suffered perinatal losses. Chronic sorrow, or "shadow grief," is a way of coming to terms with a changed, sometimes suffering self.

Shadow grief is a form of chronic grief and does not manifest itself overtly. It does not debilitate; no effort is required to cope with it. On the surface most observers would say that the grief work has been accomplished. But this is not the case. Shadow grief reveals itself more in the form of an emotional dullness, in which the person is unable to respond fully and completely to outer stimulation and in which normal activity is moderately inhibited. We found this to be true of some of the survivors in this study. They characterized their grief as a dull ache in the background of their feelings that remained fairly constant and that, under certain circumstances and on certain occasions, came bubbling to the surface, sometimes in the form of tears, sometimes not, but always accompanied by a feeling of sadness and a mild sense of anxiety. Individuals who experience shadow grief can never remember the events surrounding the loss without feeling some kind of emotional reaction, regardless of how mild.

After reviewing various models, the research literature and clinical experiences, the Committee for the Study of Health Consequences of the Stress of Bereavement (Osterweis, Solomon and Green, 1984) concluded that there was no clear fixed endpoint for the grieving process, that for many the process continued for a lifetime, and that there can be adjustment to the loss without a complete ending to the process or withdrawal of attachment to the deceased.

MODEL OF NORMAL BEREAVEMENT

Normal grief following the death of a loved one may continue for a lifetime even though the survivor has adjusted to the loss and recovered everyday functioning. While most grievers lessen their ties to the deceased over the first two years, it is not the length of time that separates normal from abnormal reactions. One must examine the quality and quantity of these reactions. Some of the initial tasks the bereaved goes through are: shock, anguish, mourning and, finally, recovery.

Most of the models and explanations of the grieving process over the past twenty years are derived from the work of Freud (1917) and Lindemann (1944). Bowlby (1960) and Parkes (1972) will be used to provide a detailed descriptive account of the normal phases of the grief process, which include the following classical elements: (l) shock and numbness; (2) yearning and searching; (3) disorientation and disorganization; and (4) resolution and re-organization.

Shock and Numbness

Numbness or denial is the first response on learning of the death. The survivor may respond with a refusal to accept or comprehend the fact, often crying out, "No! It can't be!" The person may throw herself or himself on the body, attempting to find signs of life or to bring the dead back to life.

This is a time when the bereaved person's usual coping strategies are overwhelmed. It is also a period of time out—a time for preparing to deal with the trauma. For many survivors these issues will be sorted out after the first few weeks, and the reaction to the death or deaths will appear. During this time the ego defense mechanism of denial shields the person from the full impact of the death; however, the effectiveness of this defense usually diminishes as more and more intrusions of reality (attending the funeral, sitting shiva, going to a memorial service) are experienced and acknowledged.

Many may try desperately, but in an automatic fashion, to carry on their ordinary activities, as if nothing had happened. Or they may sit motionless and dazed, unable to move. At such times, the survivor seems out of contact, and it may be difficult to gain her/his attention. This phase may last a few minutes or hours or even days, alternating with flashes of despair and anguish as the reality of the loss briefly penetrates the consciousness.

Sometimes, the initial response is overtly an intellectual acceptance of the reality of the loss and an immediate initiation of apparently appropriate activity, such as making arrangements and comforting others. It is only by not permitting access to consciousness of the full emotional impact of the loss that appropriate activity can take place. Although the loss is recognized, its painful nature is denied to some degree or at least muted.

Distinctive of this initial phase are the attempts to protect oneself against the effects of the overwhelming stress by raising the threshold against its recognition or against the painful feelings being evoked. Although such responses are more usual and more intense when the death is sudden and unexpected, they may also be observed even when the death has been anticipated.

Yearning and Searching

This phase is characterized by a rise in the level of affect. Once the numbing fades the next responses are those of intense distress at being separated from the deceased. There is yearning and longing for the loved one to return, to not be dead. The bereaved hopes for reunion, and looks everywhere for the deceased. The yearning and searching is most pronounced when the survivor returns to familiar environments, such as the home or places that were shared with the deceased. In strange or different environments, such as the hospital where the deceased may have been cared for, a theatre or the homes of friends that the bereaved visited with the deceased, the yearning and longing may be accompanied by a feeling that the deceased is present. The yearning and longing are accompanied by waves of intense physical distress, including breathing difficulties, palpitations, weakness and epigastic discomfort. The pain is felt internally, and may be experienced as if some physical part of the body has been lost or torn away (Raphael 1983).

The beginning of what has been called "separation pain" is expressed in tearfulness and sobbing, angry outbursts, restlessness, tension, irritability, intense yearning for the absent loved one and panic. This is an extremely stressful period that eventually affects one's self-perception, living patterns and social relationships. There is anxiety about experiencing this anguish, a sense of disorganization in terms of living arrangements and an obsessional review of the circumstances related to the death.

Anger may erupt toward persons or circumstances held to be responsible for the death—the doctor, hospital or other family members. The survivor may feel a sense of failure and may berate or even impulsively injure her/himself. Beating the breast, pounding the head or thrusting a fist through glass are occasional impulsive, aggressive and self-destructive acts on the part of the person who is suddenly overwhelmed with grief. Changes in sleeping and eating habits and energy levels are exhibited. Aches and pains may develop, as well as periods of intense disturbance followed by periods of calm. Blocking of feelings, partial disbelief, inhibitions of painful thoughts and evocation of pleasant memories are used to lessen the impact of these stressful reactions.

Crying seems to involve both an acknowledgment of the loss and a regression to a more helpless and childlike state. Grief is one situation in which the tears of an adult are generally accepted and understood, and the person who is able to cry still feels self-respect and deserving of help.

Some people want to cry or feel that they should cry, yet are unable to do so. This type of inhibition of crying must be distinguished from not crying because the person who died is not seriously missed, in which case there is no inclination or need to cry, and from the voluntary suppression of crying because of an environmental or cultural demand, in which case the person either "cries inwardly" or waits until she/he is alone and unobserved before crying. Inability to cry, however, is a more serious matter. It is most likely to occur when the relationship with the dead person was highly ambivalent and when the survivor is experiencing a good deal of guilt and shame. AIDS survivors are likely to experience some of this ambivalence, which is discussed later. This second phase of yearning and searching seems to peak two to four weeks after the loss but continues, with varying intensity, for three months or longer.

Disorientation and Disorganization

This phase represents giving up the search for the deceased. Depression and a lack of interest in the future are typical features of this period. Although images of the deceased intrude into the consciousness, they may bring a different sort of pain. For the most part, the image is in place of reality, and it is when the dead person is not available that the pain is felt. The images of the death scene itself may intrude in instances where the survivor has experienced a personal and traumatic encounter with the death. The bereaved may try to avoid reminders of the person or may attempt to repress the feelings of longing, anxiety and anger that are so painful.

Various patterns of physical and emotional distress become evident. Physical symptoms of stress appear. Complaints may vary from cold symptoms, flu, tiredness and insomnia to a range of psychosomatic illnesses. Physical responses include gastrointestinal problems, sleep disturbances, respiratory changes, fatigue, overactivity and restlessness. Psychological manifestations may include preoccupation with the deceased, time disorientation and an inability to concentrate or take the initiative in social situations (Gauthier & Marshall 1977). Physicians, without a careful assessment, may diagnose the symptoms as clinical depression, rather than part of the mourning process. In treating bereaved survivors physicians often prescribe drugs.

Contrary to popular belief, antidepressants and tranquilizers are not appropriate for treatment except in rare circumstances. Drugs may mask the symptoms and lead to a long-term unresolved grief reaction.

Drugs that are calming or anesthetizing are nontherapeutic, in that they keep the griever from experiencing the pain and realizing the loss that ultimately has to be faced. Often the bereaved are drugged during the wake and funeral, the precise times at which they should be encouraged to give vent to their emotions. This leaves them to confront their loss later on, at times in which there may not be the social support that is usually available during the initial period following the death (Rando 1984).

Although heavy sedation to block the mourning process is not wise, mild sedation to prevent exhaustion and severe insomnia, and disease resulting from them, may be quite therapeutic and necessary.

C. S. Lewis (1981) describes this period of disorganization where progress is slow and transition from one phase to another is not usually distinct. Expressions of despair, distress, anxiety, irritability and guilt are evident:

Grief is like a long valley, a winding valley where any bend may reveal a totally new landscape. As I've already noted, not every bend does. Sometimes the surprise is the opposite one; you are presented with exactly the same sort of country you thought you left behind miles ago. That is when you wonder whether the valley isn't a circular trench. But it isn't. There are partial recurrences, but the sequence doesn't repeat. (69)

This phase of disorganization and disorientation is one of the most likely periods for the contemplation of suicide by the survivor. Disorientation appears most intense from the fourth to sixth month following the death. Friends, family members and co-workers often communicate the expectation that the bereaved should be over their mourning. The survivor feels more pressure from the expectations of others, while at the same time experiencing heightened anxiety over an inability to organize thoughts and actions. The characteristics of disorganization are a necessary part of grief work and lead into progressive adaptation and integration of the loss.

Time by itself does not heal all things. The support of warm, understanding family members and friends who appreciate the bereaved person's situation and feelings can have a definite therapeutic influence. The presence of an interested, sympathetic and loving person can do more than all the tranquilizers, sleeping pills and other medicines combined to assist survivors in coping with loss and grief.

Resolution and Reorganization

During this final phase there is a gradual return of interest in the future. Attachments to the lost loved one are broken down and new ties are established with others. The survivor becomes more able to accept the finality of the loved one's death.

The past is not severed from the mourner's life, but rather the person changes in relationship to it. The gap between the past life and the future life is bridged more easily when elements of the past are incorporated into the present, but with an altered emphasis. Ways have to be found to remember, but less painfully, to provide continuity between the past and the future. The transitional period comes to an end not when a particular event occurs but rather when the questioning and exploring have lost their urgency and emphasis is given to the development of a new life structure (Levinson et al. 1978).

In this time of mourning, there is a gradual process of review, an undoing of the psychological bonds, one by one. Memories may be vivid and spontaneous, coming in flashes before the bereaved person's eyes like a motion picture. Memories can be triggered by some place or object, or by some sound, smell or sight. Things that have belonged to the dead person may take on a special symbolic significance, becoming what Volkan (1972) has called "linking objects." With the memories come a continuing range of feelings, including despair, great sadness at what is now irretrievably gone and anger at the futility of death.

The entire reorganization process can vary from individual to individual, sometimes taking several years to complete (Silverman & Copperband 1975). Increasingly longer periods of emotional stability are experienced, as well as fewer and less intense emotional reactions.

SUDDEN DEATH

In contrast to anticipated loss, which stimulates a typical bereavement response, unexpected sudden death, such as death from a heart attack, accident, suicide, murder or sudden infant death syndrome (SIDS), prevents the survivor from being prepared. This may not be the case in death from AIDS. However, significant others may be unaware of the illness of the deceased, and may hear the news immediately after the death, leaving the survivor overwhelmed with the unexpected loss. In the case of AIDS as well as in other deaths, bereavement reactions may be more severe, exaggerated and complicated when the death occurs unexpectedly. The coping mechanisms of the bereaved may be overwhelmed. The unexpected loss causes an accelerated rate of change in the environment, a factor that is itself a stressor (Rabkin & Struening 1976). The physical and psychological systems of the person may be overwhelmed by the demands placed on them. This often leads to physical distress and feelings of helplessness and depression.

Survivors responding to Rudestam's (1977) survey on suicide indicated that they felt unprepared and described the event as being "like a devastating emotional blow" (222). Seemingly, the greater the trauma, shame, guilt, insecurity and disorientation, the greater the tendency for denial, avoidance, retreat, isolation and the wish to escape. The desire for denial is understandable and justifiable. Denial serves a needed and critical purpose for a period of time. Too much reality too fast could be psychologically overwhelming to some, and to impose a reality on needed denial could be a gross treatment error (Margolis et al. 1981).

Knapp (1986) states that sudden death generates a different kind of grief—a harsher variety. His investigation of parents of dead children revealed reactions of intense shock, numbness, disbelief and total confusion. As they moved through the experience, feelings of helplessness, intense anxiety and of impending doom came into focus. These were followed by feelings of emptiness, aimlessness, hollowness. Within a short period came additional sensations of intense irritability, bitterness and gut-wrenching sadness and sorrow. Anger—intense anger—also appeared, sometimes directed at the child. Parents began to experience a loss of patterns of conduct. Interpersonal relationships became disrupted. Feelings of "coming apart" and "falling to pieces" were also common. They could find no solid ground. There was no anchorage in this wild storm that swept in from nowhere.

Physical symptoms soon appeared, taking the form of a loss of appetite or loss of sleep or constant fatigue. Somatic complaints became common: headaches, heart palpitations, stomach problems and agonizing pain in the chest. Guilt and self-blame often consumed parents throughout the entire ordeal. Later on, depression coupled with a deep sense of loneliness, accompanied by thoughts of death and self-destruction, became the mode of response (Knapp 1986).

An attempt to delay or avoid grieving is commonly reported as a primary cause of a bad response to loss. How long can one sustain the attempt to delay or avoid? Again the answer lies in the individual circumstance and case in point. It appears that occasionally someone can sustain a very long denial period with little apparent psychological maladaptation or distortion to the psyche. Parkes (1972) and Gorer (1965) conjecture that denial beyond two weeks following a death is dysfunctional. The possibility of maladaptation increases as time passes.

Lehrman (1956) finds that pathological grief reactions are more frequent when death is both sudden and unexpected. Glick, Weiss and Parkes (1974) and Parkes (1975a, 1975b) studied women who were widowed at age forty-five or younger. Those women who suffered sudden and unexpected losses developed more physical, psychological and social problems than women the same age who had anticipated their husbands' death. Flesch (1976) reports that deaths by vehicular accident or suicide pose the greatest threat to mental health because they are unexpected.

Sudden death leaves the survivor no time to work on unfinished relationship issues or to reach a sense of closure. Reactions of shock, disbelief and denial are accentuated, thereby altering the composition of the initial phases of grief work. This does not mean that grief is less painful with other types of death. The event of sudden and unexpected death is so dramatic that it defies description and demands a more complicated bereavement.

ANTICIPATORY GRIEF

Lindemann (1944) first coined the term "anticipatory grief reactions" to refer specifically to the observed grief in the face of possible death, as in the case of relatives' reactions to a member of the armed services entering combat during World War II. Aldrich (1974) extended the concept of anticipatory grief by using the term to describe any grief reactions occurring prior to a loss, as distinguished from the grief that occurred at or after the loss. He further elaborated on the differences between anticipatory grief and conventional grief by pointing to differences in both endpoints and acceleration. Although conventional grief can be prolonged, anticipatory grief has a finite endpoint dependent on external circumstances related to the anticipated loss.

Because of the prevalence of deaths following prolonged illness in both the general population and among the increasing number of AIDS sufferers, it is important to understand the responses of grieving survivors to this type of death. Learning about the potentially fatal or debilitating illness of a loved one may have a more intense impact than the subsequent death after the illness (Schucter et al. 1986). The initial emotional reactions in such circumstances are very similar to those of people whose loved one died suddenly, and include numbness, shock and disbelief, with great anguish following closely behind.

The suffering of a family undergoing the heartrending task of caring for a loved one during an illness, only to have the months of sacrifice and hope draw to an empty, despairing close with the loved one's death, is intense. During the course of the illness, the family contends with the pain and suffering of the sick person as well as with the personal hardships of caretaking, maintaining hope, supporting the loved one physically and emotionally and adjusting psychologically to the impending death.

Although it is painful to witness the day-by-day physical and mental changes wrought by the illness, there are some redeeming aspects to this experience. The time of illness can provide an opportunity to adjust to the impending death. Through the process of anticipatory grief, the end can become somewhat less debilitating for families. Anticipatory grieving may be possible only if the person is able to accept the potential death and does not completely deny its approach. This period can provide an opportunity to say goodbye—share feelings, resolve old rifts, remember and talk about the highlights of the person's life as related to the survivor.

This period of time is a last chance to demonstrate love for the person through physical and emotional caring. People who have made use of this quality time with a loved one report feelings of closure and satisfaction rather than feelings of things left unsaid or undone or of guilt or lingering hurt. Conversations and experiences can be cherished by survivors. The opportunity to say goodbye and separate from a loved one facilitates mourning. The relationship is ended in a loving way, and the dying person feels valued and feels that life has been meaningful (Weizman & Kamm 1985).

The opportunity for anticipatory grieving is vitally important, and structures the way grief and mourning behavior is usually expressed in those cases where there is time to adjust. Parkes (1975b) in his study of reactions of widows and widowers to the loss of a spouse reveals that in the "long-preparation" group, where survivors had time to anticipate the loss, there appeared to be: (1) less difficulty accepting the loss; (2) little evidence of guilt or self-blame; (3) little extreme emotional or stressful reaction at the time of death; (4) less anger; (5) far fewer depressive symptoms; (6) a greater tendency to formulate some way of handling the event that made it more real; (7) less likelihood of reacting with disbelief and shock; (8) a greater tendency to involve oneself in such after-death ceremonies as grave visits; (9) fewer problems with role functioning; and (10) less likelihood of developing a fixation on the past.

The notion of anticipatory grief suggests that prolonged illness prepares the survivor for the loss in a way that eases the grief once death occurs. The actual loss of the loved one, however, does not occur until the point of death, and for some, the prolonged period of illness intensifies the bonding between the family and ill member and thus makes the feelings of loss greater once death occurs.

THE FAMILY UNIT AS SURVIVOR

When a beloved family member dies, many complex issues must be faced. Although it is normal to grieve when a severe loss has been sustained, individual differences in the intensity and duration of the bereavement process are a function of multiple variables, including age, sex, personality, the sociocultural context, the relationship of the mourner to the deceased and whether or not the death was expected. The events of the past are usually recycled in the present, and the unresolved relationship issues in the family of origin (parents and siblings) will appear in the family of procreation (spouse and children) and family of function (individuals in one's social network). Without clarification and resolution, issues and relationships surrounding loss and death will be reactivated in the present. Thus, knowledge of the family's functioning during earlier stressful events will be a valuable aid in predicting how the family will respond to the mourning process.

Certain bereavements—that is, the loss of particular relationships—are also more difficult to resolve. For instance, the death of a child is terrible for parents. There is no doubt that the death of a child is the greatest tragedy any family can endure. The relationship between parent and child is life's most intimate bond, and an implicit part of that bond is that the elder will forever protect the younger. When young children die, parents are always left with the feeling that they should somehow have been able to protect the child, and with guilt that they survived in the child's place.

When a child dies, so do the family's hopes and dreams for the future. The shattering of a family's dreams may be particularly poignant when the child had yet to reach adulthood, for parents can only imagine what might have been. Could this child have reached beyond the parents' own achievements? The family's sense of its very future is brought into question with the loss of the next generation.

A major task of mid-life is to accept the realization that the major portion of one's life lies behind rather than ahead. Separation and loss are crucial events in the life cycle. However, the loss of a child when parents are in their forties, fifties or sixties actualizes one of our deepest fears—death before fulfillment (Moss & Moss 1983–84; Pine & Brauer 1986). Major "non-normative" losses tend to have a profound impact on parents, which upsets the rhythm of life: "The most distressing and long-lasting of all grief is that of the loss of a grown child. In such a case it seems to be literally true, and not a figure of speech, that the parents never get over it" (Gorer 1967, 72).

The relationship between a middle-aged parent and a adult child is quite different from that between a parent and younger child, and differences in the grief experience should be anticipated. It may be particularly difficult to see one's offspring denied the rewards of adulthood after years of struggle for education and job security. Also, an adult-parent relationship that has been strained or has matured over time is hard to relinquish. For the parent, developmental issues related to personal losses such as retirement, widowhood or failing health affect mourning and further complicate grieving (Dane 1990).

Widowhood has an effect on all of an individual's family relationships. If there are children in the home, the widow or widower has to play the roles of both mother and father. Although members of the extended family are usually in close contact with the widowed person for a while after the death of the spouse, interactions with them become less frequent as time passes. Widowhood is, without question, the greatest life crisis for most women and men. A widowed person loses a friend, a lover, a helpmate and a part of his/her identity as a person. The status of widowhood is usually accompanied by financial changes and often loneliness.

The death of a spouse may also make for serious problems of resolution, particularly for men who feel they should have been able to save and protect their wife. Among adult women, it has been found that emotional reactions to the loss of a husband are usually less intense in older than in younger widows. For example, Ball (1977) found that widows in the eighteen to forty-six year age bracket grieved more intensely than widows who were over age forty-six. One explanation for this age difference in grief is that in the case of an older widow, the death of her (older) husband is more likely to have been anticipated, thus providing an opportunity to prepare for it. Younger women also often have children to raise, under difficult economic circumstances.

Lopata's (1973) study found that the strength of the relationship between a married couple has a pronounced effect on the grief shown by the surviving member. The stronger the emotional bond, the more difficult the recovery process. Relationships characterized by extreme dependency or persisting conflict are indicative of a poor recovery prognosis. But when the relationship is built on mutual trust and fulfillment, the bereaved person can more easily get on with the process of readjustment and self-renewal.

Adults who are preoccupied with their own grief and with the life reorganization necessitated by the death of a spouse or other loved one sometimes overlook the fact that surviving children also experience grief and other emotions associated with death. Children who have sustained the loss of a parent or sibling in particular, as well as a close relative or friend, experience grief just as adults do, and can be quite upset and confused. A bereaved child should be permitted to ask questions and encouraged to express feelings about the death and the deceased. Adults should acknowledge the child's questions and feelings, including anger, guilt, anxiety and sadness. Negative feelings and memories should be accepted and worked through, but adults should also try to get the child to focus on happy moments that were shared with the deceased and to think about something the child did to please the deceased (Schlesinger 1971).

When the deceased is a parent or other adult who was very close to the child, the child will need to learn to redirect love toward another adult. It is important that not all the child's love be reinvested in a single individual, such as the surviving parent; otherwise, a condition of extreme dependency may develop. The child should be encouraged to establish close relationships with several adults, especially those within the family circle (Schlesinger 1971).

In general, children experience greater difficulty adjusting to the loss of a family member when intrafamilial relationships are strained (Hilgard & Newman and Fisk 1960). But children tend to work through their problems and get on with their lives more quickly than adults, for whom the loss of a friend or family member is usually more traumatic (Cohen & Ahearn 1980).

A number of studies as reported by Martin (1989) have explored how the relationship of the deceased to the bereaved has affected the course of grief. Balk (1983) focused on the effects of sibling death on teenagers. Thirty-three teenagers were interviewed, evenly divided between younger (fourteen to sixteen years old) and older (seventeen to nineteen years old). In addition, the Offer Self-Image Questionnaire for Adolescents was administered. Sibling death had occurred on average 23.6 months prior to the interview, with a range of 4 to 84 months. Grief symptoms ranged from a negative impact of the loss on school work to thoughts of suicide. Both peers and family were reported as having been helpful in alleviating the stress associated with the deaths. The results of the self-concept measure were inconclusive. Balk concluded that most of the teenagers were adjusting to their losses and had emerged from the experience as more mature individuals.

Sanders (1980) administered the Grief Experience Inventory and the Minnesota Multi-Phase Inventory MMPI to 102 newly bereaved subjects. In addition, 107 controls, matched for age and sex, were assessed. A comparison of the intensity of bereavement across three types of bereavement—death of parent, spouse and child—showed that the death of a child produced the highest intensities of bereavement.

Owen, Fulton and Markusen (1982–83) studied family survivors in the Minneapolis-St. Paul area. Data were collected using both questionnaires and home interviews from 558 bereaved persons, including 434 spouses, 85 parents and 39 adult children responding to the death of an elderly parent. Of the sample, 72% was female, 97% white; also, 47% of those interviewed lived alone.

Responses showed that the pattern of post-death adjustment for the three groups confirmed the findings reported by Sanders (1980): the type of relationship severed by death was an important determinant of the nature of the grief experienced by survivors. Results indicated that the death of an elderly parent appeared to be of limited significance to their adult child. We know that this response, however, is very individual. This was particularly true if the parent was old, of the same sex as the surviving child, and had been institutionalized prior to death. By contrast, the death of a child or spouse presented the bereaved with an intense grief experience.

Grief in nontraditional relationships such as homosexual and bisexual ones is understudied. Because these relationships are negatively sanctioned, feelings of guilt may be particularly evident. Extreme isolation, loneliness and even a deep sense of persecution (Doka 1987) may be experienced. While these relationships may differ in many ways, bereavement can be complicated since resources for resolving grief are often limited.

RELIGIOUS AND CULTURAL BELIEFS

There are social, ethnic, cultural and religious variations in the expression of emotions. Traditionally, ritual has been an important element of the leave-taking process, and funeral customs are a primary source of this ritual. Most definitions of funeral ritual, however, are generally confined to those immediately surrounding the death, beginning with the notification of death and ending with a gathering for food and social interaction after a service. Wilcox and Sutton (1977) suggest that "ritual makes sense of death by placing it in the context of a world view. . . . As the distance from one's own death increases and the right to mourn is taken away, the ability to 'make sense' of death breaks down and there is growing dissatisfaction with the ritual that supports that rationalization" (163).

As clinicians we must be knowledgeable about acceptable practices in helping survivors receive comfort from their religious and cultural beliefs. Rituals can provide powerful therapeutic experiences that symbolize transition, healing and continuity (Van der Hart 1983). Their power comes not from magic but from the faith the individual has in their ability to provide meaning.

For most individuals the religious element in the support system is significant. For those without an organized religion as a base for that support, key persons during the death process, such as clergy, can fill this role, even temporarily. More than in any other experience, those suffering acute grief need a philosophical basis for understanding and coping with their crisis. The need is there and becomes even more apparent for those who move away from institutionalized religion and a philosophy of life and death (Keith 1981).

The final element in the support system, known and repeated ceremonial forms, is still intact for most people. There are, however, repeated criticisms of contemporary funeral rituals as being meaningless and valueless for survivors. In some instances a person gives instructions to the family that she/he wants no ritual or ceremony following death.

It is erroneous to generalize that all people surviving a death need a funeral to resolve their grief. Many of the rituals of the funeral serve the important function of emphasizing clearly and unequivocally the reality of the death, the denial of which cannot be allowed to go on if recovery from the loss is to take place. The viewing of the body, the lowering of the casket and the various rituals of different religious beliefs allow for no ambiguity. Further, this experience takes place in a group, permitting ordinarily guarded feelings to be shared and expressed more readily.

The funeral experience also initiates the process of identification with the lost person through the various rituals that symbolize an identity between the mourner and the dead. In many cultures, the funeral ceremony includes a feast or some sort of wake in which are symbolically expressed a triumph over death, a denial of the fear of death or of the dead, an attempt to return to life and living (Engel 1964). Rituals do not have to be dramatic, but should be tailored to the needs of the survivor if they are to be meaningful and helpful.

Some survivors initially seem to cope with the death by turning to a religious interpretation of what happened. Parents whose child died may feel a loss of faith, with anger and sometimes even hatred toward a God who "allowed this terrible thing to happen." Parents often ask: "Why did God do this to us?" Parents cannot fathom a benevolent God allowing something terrible to happen to children. Many parents who blamed God indicated later that they did not really feel any shame for doing so, and that at the time it felt good to be able to hold someone responsible. They came to realize that God was indeed "big enough" to take it (Knapp 1986).

Despite interesting ceremonial vestiges, in contemporary society the distinguishing aspects of ethnic groups are more likely to be reflected in deep-seated beliefs than in ritual practice. Ethnic beliefs may also be at the core of unresolved family issues, and framing them in ethnic terms may help lead to resolution.

African-Americans, Puerto Ricans and most Mediterranean peoples are openly expressive of grief. African-Americans tend to have strong suspicions of "the system." Traditionally they have relied upon the kinship network, particularly embodied in women, to provide physical and emotional support in times of distress (Rosen 1990). Mourners at Puerto Rican or Iranian funerals have been known to faint from the exertion of wailing and screaming. To sit quietly at the funeral may be considered a breach of etiquette. Other ethnic groups are less likely to display their sorrow, either in public or private. The Irish wake is more like a celebration than a sad farewell, and while much emotion is expressed, it is likely to be lubricated by drink, anecdotes and humor because of the belief in an easier afterlife. Many Asian cultures greatly constrain the emotional expression of grief, but offer a highly ritualized framework for mourning. White Protestant middle-class culture neither accepts public emotional displays nor offers sanctioned outlets for emotions.

SUMMARY

The struggle to accommodate loss is a fact of life, and permeates each stage of the life cycle. It represents much of the individual's efforts to come to terms with the issue of mortality. Kalish (1985) states: "Anything you have you can lose; anything you are attached to, you can be separated from; anything you love can be taken from you. Yet, if you really have nothing to lose, you have nothing" (141).

Bereavement refers to the state of loss or deprivation that results from the death of another person. Grief is the feeling of sorrow and distress that results from bereavement. Mourning is the culturally prescribed behavior pattern for expressing grief. Enduring the transition of a loved one from life to death can be a very abrupt and devastating experience. Dane (1990) states that "the overriding issue that faces us in all our determination to cope with loss and to help others cope with loss is the place accorded to death in our lives today. Mourning is not only normal, but essential" (467).

It is hoped that numerous practical, psychological and social considerations will be accounted for in working with survivors. The role of the practitioner is vital in assisting the bereaved to cope with the death of a loved one. Death is a part of life, and an important task for practitioners is to help survivors "let go," which is rarely easy to do.

Grief has many facets, but an understanding of the process and sensitivity to individual differences is critical in meeting the needs of survivors. In our society, grief reactions are often viewed with suspicion. It is not long before the mourner is exhorted to "get on with it" or is assured that everything will be right again as soon as the mourner stops feeling sorry for her/himself. Negative reactions such as these often encourage people to bury their grief. Consequently, they do not complete the tasks of mourning and never learn to accept their losses so they can move on (Dane 1990). Understanding the concept of family balance and cultural, religious and ethnic differences in mourning can provide the mourners with support as they experience confusion, pain and emptiness.

As with other aspects of trauma, there is a sense of having to continue with life. Most people have some hope of things getting better, of recovery, of trust in life and love that again draws them on into the future. Professionals can give license to start anew, but they must also be very careful not to be perceived as pushing too hard or too fast before the necessary grieving has occurred.

Implicit in this discussion and the literature is the notion to "do something" with grief. Clearly, an emphasis on grief work is a good thing. Assuming, however, that one mourning style suits everyone does not do justice to the importance of individual differences. Of all the factors affecting the survivor's grief, there is none so important as the meaning of the event to the individual.

CHAPTER 2

Overview of the AIDS Crisis

Although the current epidemic of human immuno-deficiency virus (HIV) infection was officially recognized on June 5, 1981, in many respects we are just beginning to appreciate the sobering consequences of its impact. Acquired immune-disease syndrome (AIDS) has created a new agenda of public health concerns throughout the world, and perhaps nowhere more conspicuously than in the United States.

The statistics are staggering. Worldwide, an estimated 7.5 million people may be infected with the HIV virus, which is believed to be the cause of AIDS. Of those infected, 1.3 to 2.7 million are in the United States (Centers for Disease Control 1990). A recent report indicates that the number of diagnosed cases in the United States has reached 161,073 with 100,777 deaths. The number of cases, infected through various sources, has expanded exponentially since 1981 (see Figure 2.1). The World Health Organization predicts that by the year 2000 about 40 million people will be infected with the AIDS virus (Kolata 1991).

Based on cumulative reports from 149 countries through June of 1988, the world has had 157,191 cases of AIDS and between five million and ten million people are presently infected with HIV, the causative viral agent. While Asia and Oceania have thus far largely been spared, Europe, Africa, North America and South America have all been significantly affected (see Table 2.1). Preliminary evaluation of the effect of such infection rates in developing countries suggests that AIDS is so serious a threat that it may substantially reduce their population growth rates over the next few decades (Mann 1989).

The United States and central Africa have been the hardest hit, forming two epicenters of the pandemic (Figure 2.1), with 204 reported cases of AIDS per million inhabitants in the United States. In Uganda alone the numbers

Figure 2.1
U.S. AIDS Cases—The Numbers (by Year of Diagnosis)

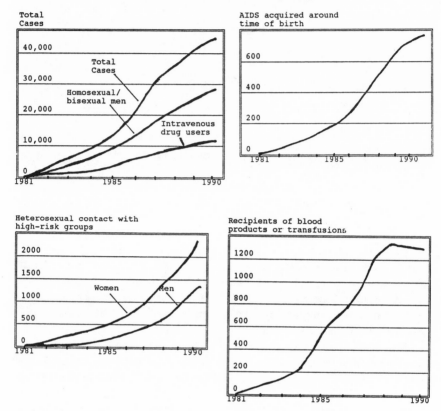

Figures are adjusted for reporting delays.

Source: Centers for Disease Control

are chilling. The bleakest prognosis, if the epidemic continues at its present rate and no efforts are made to halt it, is that instead of having a population of thirty-two million in the year 2015, Uganda will have only twenty million people. Another wrenching statistic is that five to six million Ugandan children will be orphans by 2011 because their parents will have died of AIDS (*New York Times*, 1991).

Although we have made important discoveries—for example, we know what causes AIDS, and we know how it is transmitted—the impact and the prospects are worse than anyone could have imagined. AIDS has taken on the dimensions of an epidemic and has forced America to come to grips with some grim realities. Researchers persist in their attempts to develop effective medical treatments to reduce the suffering of those who are presently HIV-

Table 2.1
Reported and Estimated AIDS Cases, June 1989

Area	Cumulative Reported	number of countries	Estimated
Africa	24,686	47	270,000
Americas	108,830	43	175,000
Asia	369	24	1,000
Europe	21,855	28	32,000
Oceania	1,451	7	2,000
TOTAL	157,191	149	480,000

Source: Mann 1989, 9

infected or seriously ill with full-blown AIDS. Despite research efforts, there are no vaccines against AIDS, no cures for it and few effective treatments. It is clear that many people will suffer prolonged, expensive and untimely deaths as a result of the immune damage wrought by this viral infection.

As the AIDS epidemic begins its second decade, practitioners, researchers and advocates for people with the ailment have all painfully abandoned their once keen hopes of bringing the scourge quickly under control. Researchers say that they are settling in for the long haul, expecting the battle against AIDS to occupy the rest of their working lives.

Advocates say that they are trying to decide where to focus their energies and how to maintain the nation's flagging interest in the dread disease. Some advocates say that they are finding it hard to keep their spirits up. "Morale is exceptionally low," notes Larry Kramer (1991), founder of the AIDS Coalition to Unleash Power/ACT UP. "People are living longer, but after ten years we perceive that very little progress has been made. We thought we could change the world if we could just become part of the system, getting ourselves seats on crucial federal committees. But now we have learned that is not enough."

In this chapter, we will focus on the evolution of AIDS, its transmission, the populations susceptible to high-risk behaviors, the politics and the fears and stigma associated with AIDS. While a great deal has been learned about AIDS over the past ten years, much is still unknown, and even less is understood, about the invisible survivors of persons who have died of AIDS. In this overview, we will present the findings that have thrown some light on this tragedy of AIDS and that help us to understand how it is perceived and managed by survivors of people who have died from AIDS in our contemporary society.

EVOLUTION OF AIDS AS A CRISIS AND ILLNESS

Of all the viruses that have plagued human beings through the ages, few have cast darker shadows or proved more formidable than the one that causes AIDS. AIDS is a life-threatening condition characterized by a serious impairment of the cell-mediated branch of the immune system, which leaves the person defenseless against infections and certain forms of malignancies. The two diseases most commonly found in AIDS patients are pneumocystis carinii pneumonia, a lung infection caused by a parasite, and Karposi's sarcoma, a rare form of cancer of the blood vessels. Other diseases, notably tuberculosis, hepatitis, neurological diseases, herpes, AIDS dementia, blindness and neuropathy, accompany AIDS and impair and isolate PWAs long before finally killing them. Experimental treatments with some antiviral agents have proven to delay the onset of symptoms in HIV-positive individuals and to prolong the lives of PWAs. Nevertheless, the mortality rate of AIDS patients is 100% (Valdiserri, Tama & Ho 1988).

The population of persons with AIDS includes, among others, individuals who live in family structures that parallel the traditional nuclear family (e.g., homosexual couples and unmarried couples in long-term relationships). In many ways they retain distinctive characteristics, including the lack of legal and social sanction, that significantly influence the quality of life of their members. The impact of AIDS affects both the person with AIDS and their invisible survivors: families, lovers, friends and significant others. AIDS, like any illness, affects the entire family system. Individual and family members have to live day after day with the deadly consequences of the infectious human immunodeficiency virus.

Since AIDS was first identified, it has been the subject of intense medical, epidemiological, political, religious, economic and social controversy. AIDS was presumably introduced into the United States in the 1970s, but was not recognized clinically until 1981. Although it is not absolutely certain whether the HIV-induced syndrome is a new disease, or where it came from, serologic data are now accumulating that suggest that the disease existed in Africa at least a decade before it came to the United States, probably via Haiti (Gonda 1986). Scientists have found an animal virus, STV-III (simian T-lymphotropic virus type III), which causes an AIDS-like syndrome in the macaque monkey and may have given rise to a human variant such as AIDS. Moreover, antibodies to the AIDS virus exist in the blood of otherwise healthy African green monkeys (Rodway & Wright 1988).

In 1980, the Centers for Disease Control noted an unusual cluster of deaths secondary to pneumocystis pneumonia and Karposi's sarcoma among homosexual men (Ron & Rogers 1989). The early cases had in common a large number of sexual contacts, many with traceable contacts to each other. Not long thereafter, intravenous drug users were also found to be coming down with pneumocystis pneumonia. Soon it was evident that the disease was caused by a filterable agent, probably transmitted in a manner similar to hepatitis B, by blood or through sexual contact.

By 1984, the virus had been identified, the profound immunosuppression of patients with AIDS had been recognized, serologic methods had been developed to detect the HIV antibody, the clinical syndromes resulting from HIV infection had become well defined and the opportunistic infections most commonly seen in conjunction with the infection had been identified. There was hope that drugs to treat AIDS and a vaccine to prevent it would soon follow (Ron & Rogers 1989).

With no quick technological fix, the public has become uneasy, and its response filled with conflicting currents: "scientific ineptitude explains the absence of a vaccine, while others propose that scientists have been malignly sluggish in their efforts due to bias against the socially peripheral groups who comprise a large proportion of the number of persons with AIDS" (Osborn 1989, 124). From the outset AIDS has been associated with illicit intimacy—it is a "dirty disease" (Freidland 1989).

The magnitude of the AIDS epidemic and the urgency of developing a variety of appropriate treatments or a cure present an enormous challenge for medical research. AIDS, more than any other disease, has raised a host of complex questions, from those concerning the most fundamental nature of biological systems to those concerning the role of scientific research in society at large.

Beyond the challenge to biomedical research, there are profound and broader implications of the AIDS crisis for every sector of the health care provision system and, consequently, for every member of the health care team, both personally and professionally. AIDS may ultimately become a serious chronic disease, not totally unlike others that now exist and that are susceptible to drug and other proven therapies. In the interim, however, we live with a disease that is incurable, that clearly has a long incubation period and is lodged in millions throughout the world who will one day show the symptoms of their condition. There is a growing sense of anxiety about the future. AIDS is with us despite our resistance to accept the disease.

THE COURSE OF TRANSMISSION

The primary means of HIV transmission is by blood and by direct contact of genital or rectal mucosa with infected semen or vaginal secretions. Although HIV may be found in virtually any body fluid, only blood, semen and vaginal or cervical secretions are thought to be important in viral transmission. HIV has been detected in saliva and tears, but there is no evidence that the virus is transmitted through these fluids (Corless & Lindeman 1988).

HIV is transmitted only through the intimate exchange of body fluids, specifically semen, vaginal fluid, blood and mother's milk. The activities identified with a high risk of the transmission of HIV are anal, oral and vaginal sex, the use of infected blood or blood products, the sharing of infected drug paraphernalia, and breastfeeding. HIV is also transmitted from mother to fetus in the uterus or during birth (Mass 1987; Heyward & Curran 1989). The risk of acquiring HIV infection from a single sexual encounter with an infected person remains unknown at this time (Freidland & Klein 1987), yet infection can occur from a single sexual contact (Mann 1989).

Health care workers have been concerned about the risks of occupational infection with HIV. Researchers who studied surgical procedures at San Francisco General Hospital, which serves a population that is at a very high risk for AIDS, say that, on average, one surgeon or operating room nurse every eight years will be infected with the AIDS virus on the job (Altman 1990). Some surgeons have demanded that patients be tested for the AIDS virus before surgery to alert doctors and nurses to be especially careful in the operating room. The same report found that testing for the AIDS virus before surgery would not reduce the frequency of accidental exposure to blood in the operating room.

A Florida dentist who died from AIDS was known to have infected five patients with the same strain of the AIDS virus, after performing invasive procedures on them. As of late 1991, the case of this dentist is the only known one in which the AIDS virus was transmitted from a health care worker to a patient out of more than 175,000 AIDS cases reported since the disease was discovered in 1981. New findings may intensify pressure on federal officials to issue guidelines for health care workers regarding testing for AIDS (*New York Times* 1991).

Persons providing mental health care for persons with AIDS or HIV infection are generally at lower risk for HIV infection due to patient contact than is the case with medical personnel. Nevertheless, there are mental health professionals who do work in settings where exposure to blood and other potentially infectious body fluids does occur. For example, persons working with the developmentally disabled, in child-care institutions, in drug treatment settings, in prisons and in psychiatric institutions may find themselves in situations where blood or other body fluids are spilled. In such cases, the infection control practices advocated for medical personnel are advisable.

UNSUBSTANTIATED TRANSMISSION

Other suspected modes of transmission, such as casual contact, insect bites, kissing, saliva, sweat and toilet seats, have been shown not to transmit HIV infection. There is no evidence of household transmission. Studies involving over four hundred family members of HIV-infected individuals have found no evidence of transmission to members of the household who were not sexually involved with the infected individual (Rogers 1988). People living with persons with AIDS, sharing their bathrooms and eating utensils, and hugging and kissing them at frequent intervals have not developed AIDS as a result of household contact (Freidland & Klein 1987).

POPULATIONS AT RISK

There is a danger when identifying populations at risk for HIV-AIDS because people not in these groups will see themselves as separate from the problem. As a result, both knowledge of and systematic reflection on the interaction of biological, psychological, social, economic, political and cultural factors will be minimized. For our discussion, however, it should be noted that the impact of AIDS is disproportionately high in groups that have on a societal level been powerless and stigmatized. AIDS has clearly changed from a decade ago when it was discovered and the epidemic was thought to involve primarily gay and bisexual men. The prevalence of HIV is growing rapidly among intravenous drug abusers and their sexual partners and newborns.

By the year 2000, there will be ten million cases of AIDS worldwide, 90% of them in developing countries, principally among the impoverished. At the June 1991 international AIDS meeting in Florence, Italy, Dr. Chin, a World Health Organization official, stated that "increasingly, heterosexual transmission will become the predominant mode of HIV transmission throughout the world," and that women will account for increasing numbers of cases (Altman, 1991). The expectation is that the AIDS infection will spread more widely among people who have sexually transmitted diseases.

Heterosexual transmission is expected to account for up to 70% of the infections, and homosexual transmission for about 10%. Intravenous drug users will account for 10%. (These figures, including those of infected children, will exceed 100% because of overlapping in the categories.) There are now about half a million children who have AIDS because of transmission of the virus from their mothers in pregnancy. By the year 2000, about ten million children will be orphaned. Examining the populations that have had the heaviest concentration of HIV infection broadens our perspective on the impact of this epidemic.

HOMOSEXUAL AND BISEXUAL MEN

The largest group, which accounts for 65% of all adult AIDS cases, is homosexual and bisexual men. The ages of highest risk are twenty-five to forty-four years. Gay men who are also intravenous drug users account for approximately 8% of additional AIDS cases, while heterosexual intravenous drug users represent approximately 17% of AIDS cases. The issues of homosexual and bisexual men, including factors related to transmission, will be discussed more extensively in Chapters 6 and 8.

HEMOPHILIACS

Hemophiliacs (1%), other persons with a history of blood transfusion (2%), and individuals who contracted AIDS during heterosexual activities (4%) represent other populations at risk (Centers for Disease Control 1986). The incidence of HIV infection among persons with hemophilia is difficult to determine, due to this population's reluctance to be tested for the presence of antibodies. The Centers for Disease Control estimate that up to 92% of those with hemophilia A and up to 52% of those with hemophilia B have been infected with HIV (Stehr-Green, Holman, Jason & Evatt 1988).

WOMEN

A 1991 study reports a disproportionate increase in cases of AIDS over the past three years among women who are heterosexual partners of bisexual men (16%) or heterosexual partners of intravenous drug users (67%). From 1981 to 1986 reported cases of AIDS in women increased in parallel with cases in men. Although men with AIDS still dramatically outnumber women with AIDS, it is noteworthy that the proportion of women with AIDS, whose only risk factor was heterosexual contact with someone at risk, increased from 12% in 1982 to 26% in 1986 (Guinan & Hardy 1987). Public Health Service projections estimate that by 1992, between 25,000 and 31,000 women will be diagnosed with AIDS (Murphy 1988).

Women with AIDS have more trouble obtaining government disability payments than do men with AIDS because the standard definition of AIDS does not take into account many of the symptoms experienced by women. For example, health agencies list Karposi's sarcoma, an AIDS-related cancer, as part of the definition, but some experts say women with AIDS rarely get this type of cancer. Cervical cancer, on the other hand, is not now part of the definition. To date, if a woman is HIV-positive and has had bouts of bacterial pneumonia, the beginnings of cervical cancer, pelvic inflammatory disease and a severely depleted immune system she does not automatically qualify. A long ordeal of application and appeal can take several years. Women on average die of AIDS in half the time of men with the disease, although researchers do not know why this is so.

Prostitutes and their partners are at increased risk of exposure to AIDS. Many of these women feel that the risk must be accepted in order to survive financially. In Nevada and Los Angeles, all prostitutes are regularly tested. This was defended on the grounds that prostitution cannot be eliminated, and that safety may be increased through regulation. These approaches address the risk posed to the customer by infected prostitutes but fail to offer any protection to the prostitutes themselves.

Women with AIDS pose further complex problems. Researchers have found that trends in women with AIDS are good predictors of trends in pediatric AIDS cases, especially among mothers in identifiable risk groups (Guinan & Hardy 1987). In approximately 65% of the pregnancies of women who are infected with the virus, infection is passed on to the infant, and close to 50% of those infants will have AIDS within two years. The outlook for these children is almost certain death (Koop 1987; Ledger 1987).

About two-thirds of pediatric AIDS cases are the result of transmission from infected mother to child (Koop 1987). The mother may predecease the child, meaning that the sick children are also orphans. More important, not only women with AIDS but also women with HIV infection and women who are asymptomatic carriers of HIV infection have the potential to transmit the virus perinatally. HIV infection can be passed from mother to infant in three ways: to the fetus in utero through fetal-maternal circulation, to the infant during labor and delivery and possibly to the infant through infected breast milk (Freidland & Klein 1987; Curran and Jaffe 1985).

LATENCY-AGE CHILDREN

The lowest incidence of HIV infection is among latency-age children. Most children acquire the disease through perinatal transmission, and die before school age. Although there is clear evidence that transmission by casual contact does not occur, mainstreaming of school-age children with HIV infection poses a problem in many communities, reflecting the stigma and discrimination that accompany this disease.

The most vulnerable latency-age risk group is children who may have been sexually abused by an infected male. HIV transmission as a consequence of child sexual abuse has been reported. It is unknown exactly how many adolescents with AIDS may have contracted HIV as a result of sexual abuse during latency. Disorganized families on drugs may be unable to protect their young children from incest and sexual exploitation. In geographic areas with high seropositivity, sexual abuse should be considered a high-risk circumstance.

ADOLESCENTS

There is a growing awareness of the threat that the AIDS epidemic poses for adolescents. Currently, adolescents represent less than 1% of all diagnosed cases of AIDS in the United States (Centers for Disease Control 1988). However, the number of AIDS cases presently reported among adolescents is problematic and may severely underestimate the potential threat of infection as well as seroprevalence in this age-group. Considering the long and variable latency period (Curran and Jaffe 1985), and the possible time interval from infection to the appearance of symptoms, one may assume that many young adults between the ages of twenty to twenty-four acquired HIV infection as teenagers. More appropriate markers for projecting the future rate of HIV infection in the adolescent population may be the prevalence of sexual activity and rates of other sexually transmitted diseases and unintended pregnancies.

INTRAVENOUS DRUG USERS

Among high-risk groups, intravenous (IV) drug users are perhaps the most marginal figures in the AIDS epidemic. Most intravenous drug users are African-American or Hispanic. Many of them live in poverty on the edges of urban life. They fill the prisons and jails and are usually described as weak-willed, pleasure-seeking hedonists, unable to control themselves, willing to do anything for a fix, unreliable when offered treatment (Gagnon 1983).

If the epidemic maintains its present course in the United States, it is most likely to become primarily a disease of the poor and oppressed groups, populations already burdened by many health and social problems. Gay males (IV) drug users, who were stigmatized even before the AIDS epidemic, will continue to experience stigmatization. The disease will take its devastating toll.

Viewed from the perspective of suffering, AIDS not only is a menace to those afflicted with the disease but to families and intimates, to neighborhoods, to practitioners and to institutions who care for PWAs and, finally, to the rest of society. We all feel threatened by perceived sources of the epidemic, and many are profoundly affected as survivors of its consequences. The greatest chance to lessen this epidemic lies in working with targeted populations at risk and educating the entire population to reshape their lives.

POLITICS OF AIDS

The horror of the AIDS disease that claims thousands of lives demands an aggressive political and social response. Powerful responses have been evoked throughout the eleven-year history of the AIDS epidemic. Conservative political groups continue to see the occurrence of AIDS as an opportunity to prove that the moral fabric of the country is coming apart. For homosexuals, AIDS has become an important rallying cry, and they are finding in the anguish of AIDS a rebirth of the political strength they first discovered in the 1970s. Gay leaders have sought to keep the disease on the public agenda, fought for funds to treat and care for AIDS patients, and struggled for research resources necessary to understand and cope with the infection.

Several components of our social policy need to be framed in a more tolerant and flexible posture if the spread of HIV is to be reduced. Innovative changes in the policies that we have embraced for so long are needed in the areas of treatment and education. The entire political dynamics of the AIDS catastrophe are beyond the scope of this chapter, but some stark issues demand action and are highlighted. The following discussion views AIDS as a global problem, dealing with recurrent themes in public health policy despite the diversity of people and cultural mores.

The AIDS virus competes with humankind for a niche in the world. Getzel (1990) suggests that those who do not have AIDS and who perceive themselves as being in no danger of becoming HIV-infected may challenge the use of resources for people with AIDS because of the high economic and social costs. In short, compassionate concern may decrease because of self-interest and a protectionist outlook in the general population.

How the global community copes and adapts to the AIDS epidemic will serve as a model for future phases of the disease. Much has been written about the public health establishment and its failure to intervene in a timely and sensitive manner when the AIDS epidemic was first identified (Shilts 1987; Sontag 1989). Bureaucratic ineptitude and infighting and negative social attitudes abound in addressing a disease whose principal early targets were gay men. The result was resistance to approaching all issues regarding AIDS.

Early in the epidemic, scientists, the press and the public seemed curiously fixated on the origins of the virus and its possible African roots. Although this early preoccupation with Africa and Haiti as the source of the epidemic no longer dominate the scene, suspicion and mistrust continue (Airhihenbuwa 1989).

In the middle of 1982, scientists first noted that AIDS had a link to blood transfusions. Three cases had been identified among hemophiliacs who, because of their disease, are heavily dependent on the use of blood products. As noted earlier, the disease was concentrated among male homosexuals and intravenous drug users. Some federal officials saw in AIDS a pattern similar to that observed in hepatitis B, a blood-transmitted disease that is endemic in the same populations and that is a serious hazard of transfusions. Federal officials expressed their fear to representatives of several blood-banking organizations that the blood supply was being contaminated (Clark 1986). Since transmission through transfusions placed people at risk, significant improvements in the overall quality of blood services were necessary, and were finally achieved.

The likelihood of a connection between drug use and AIDS was supported by the government (Turner, Mailer & Moses 1989). One of the strongest indictments of our social policy toward both illicit drug users and people with AIDS is our low investment in treatment. Although treatment works slowly and is addressed to maintenance rather than a cure, there has been a continuing reduction in public investment in treatment for all groups, and particularly little for cocaine users (Shaffer & Jones 1989).

The largest proportion of intravenous drug users are the inner-city poor, African-American and Hispanic adults whose health, security and life chances are greatly diminished even before they are HIV-infected. Poor-quality medical services, lack of access to care and community distrust and suspicion effectively deprive inner-city people of required preventive, acute and long-term health care. Prejudice toward addicts on the part of providers and the public is accompanied by racial, ethnic and class hostilities (Getzel 1990).

Despite the deadliness of this virus, the moral fervor that demands that treatment be done in the "right" way, that is, without condoning drug use, has restricted innovative programs that would offer users bleach, clean needles or methadone. The city of San Francisco program, with its straight health message "Use bleach and stop the spread of AIDS," is one that seems to be working (Newmeyer 1988).

There have been a number of signs that public attitudes toward the disease have changed. According to a 1991 *New York Times*/CBS News poll, for example, half of American adults who are single and under forty-five years of age say they have changed their sexual behavior because of fear of getting AIDS. The most frequently cited changes were the use of condoms and limiting the number of sexual partners (Kagay 1991).

"The public is better informed about AIDS, and those at greater risk are more likely to say they have changed their sexual behavior." The poll showed support for educating children about AIDS in the schools even during the elementary school years. For instance, 42% of those polled said that they thought the schools were giving children "too little information about AIDS" (Kagay 1991).

Despite increasing public media attention to AIDS, widespread public fear, hostility and intolerance toward people with AIDS and their survivors remain. Only 39% of respondents in the poll said that they have a lot or some sympathy for "people who get AIDS from homosexual activity," and 30% said they have some sympathy for "people who get AIDS from sharing needles while using illegal drugs" (Kagay 1991). Renewed efforts to develop well-targeted, unequivocal and explicit educational messages free of moral arguments need to be designed to inform the public and promote behavioral changes as well as to sensitize the public toward the consequences of their discrimination and bigotry.

A new social policy for AIDS that reduces the spread of AIDS and encompasses white, middle-class, homosexual or bisexual groups, as well as women, children and drug users, the latter from predominantly lower-class and oppressed communities, needs to be quickly embraced to stop the excruciating deaths from AIDS. In the first years of the epidemic, the federal government did very little to fund risk reduction education. A 1989 report underscored the nature of the government's failure:

Because no vaccine is likely to become available in the near future and because of the seriousness of the disease, the only prudent course of action is an immediate major effort to stop the further spread of infection through public health measures, particularly education. Any delay will bequeath to future policy makers a problem of potentially catastrophic proportions and will condemn many thousands of individuals to infection and death. Faced with the enormity of the epidemic's potential toll, past and current efforts could only be described as woefully inadequate (Christakis 1989, 127–28).

The AIDS pandemic provides a new opportunity to view health as an international phenomenon, one that is best addressed by policies with international dimensions. AIDS demands monetary expenditure that nations have good reason to want to limit. Because every nation has an interest in the health of its citizens, an interest in AIDS control is related to a country's survival. AIDS has threatened the social structure of society and has raised troubling questions regarding thorny issues of sexual behavior, privacy rights, discrimination and professional responsibility (Christakis 1989).

In countries throughout the world, AIDS has been problematic for the insurance industry, blood-bank services, the military, the penal system and the school system. Adequately confronting the problem by utilizing a collaborative international effort requires a fostering of cooperation in AIDS control. Presently, there is a serious underreporting of AIDS cases, for a number of political and logistical reasons. Scientific information such as seroprevalence studies, case surveillance and pharmaceutical trials depend heavily on cooperation. Mistrust among nations will continue to hamper the international interest in AIDS control. In all probability, AIDS will never be eradicated, and will become a permanent part of the international agenda, like pollution and arms control. Promoting complementary ways of designing global health programs to curtail AIDS while respecting differences in the cultural conception of illness, sex and medicine can make a profound difference in the lives of persons with AIDS, their surviving family members and the international social and medical community.

Debates over the wisdom of enacting domestic AIDS quarantine laws have prompted similar debates over whether individuals should have to prove that they are AIDS-free before being allowed to engage in international travel. One of the measures some countries have taken to control the spread of the HIV is a restriction on international travel. Some have passed laws requiring certificates of HIV-free status before a person is admitted into the country; others require testing within a specified period after entry; and others test only long-term residents. In all cases either entry is denied or an alien is expelled if found seropositive (Kiapi 1989).

The United States government came under the sharp attack at the seventh international meeting on AIDS in Florence during the summer of 1991 for its policy on restricting entry of travelers infected with the disease. How to reconcile the rights of the people to cross borders freely with the duty of the state to prevent the spread of a contagious and infectious disease is a matter that has exercised the minds of nations since states system began. Officially the majority of the world community appears to be against the screening of international travellers. For example, one of the resolutions of the Forty-First World Health Assembly urged member states "to protect the human rights and dignity of HIV-infected people and people with AIDS and of members of the population groups and to avoid discriminatory action against and stigmatization of them in the provision of services, employment and travel" (Kiapi 1989, 24).

It is difficult to think of AIDS or any disease being connected to politics. We tend to think and speak of diseases in medical, physical, social, spiritual or religious terms, but not in political terms. Yet since its appearance over a decade ago, AIDS has been a political disease.

Dennis Altman, in *AIDS in the Mind of America* (1986), outlines four factors that set AIDS apart from other epidemics and help explain why this disease has been so politicized:

First, it has occurred at a time when modern medicine was believed to be well on the way to abolishing epidemic diseases altogether, at least in the Western world.

Second, it is the specific groups AIDS has affected, above all, male homosexuals. Unlike other major epidemics, of which polio is the most recent, AIDS is not seen as threatening the entire population. This attitude has begun to change, with growing evidence of heterosexual transmission.

Third, AIDS is firmly linked with sex, although this is not the only way it can be transmitted. Except for syphilis before the discovery of antibiotics, no life-threatening illness has had the potential of AIDS to be linked so clearly to sexuality and personal behavior.

Fourth, while AIDS seemed at first to be a disease primarily confined to male homosexuals, so, too, it seemed largely an American disease, and even the increasing likelihood that its origins lay in central Africa did little to shake this image. In Britain, there was a strong tendency to blame AIDS on "homosexuals who have been on 'sex holidays' to America," and a popular belief among gay men persisted for some time that one ran no risk if one confined one's sexual partners to those who had never been to North America. (80)

Just as AIDS worries individuals, it tests our health care system, our policy process and indeed, our democracy. No critical dimension of American social, professional and political life will remain untouched. In the annals of medicine, cures for diseases have come through one person's inspiration, or years of research by teams of scientists. But never have researchers or mental health professionals, working alone or together, had to struggle against the conditions that surround much of AIDS work in this country: hate, bigotry, vendettas, rage and contempt. The ugly behavior that enmesh AIDS work took root almost from the moment the AIDS epidemic was discovered over a decade ago (Rosenthal 1990).

In the beginning, fear was the soil for the anger and the fury. AIDS came so quickly, struck so hard and was so deadly. Who would not be afraid? But fear was nourished by prejudice against those who were seen then to be the only carriers of and sufferers from the disease—male homosexuals. Brand them, put them in concentration camps, are reactions rarely heard anymore but remaining in the memory.

Then it developed that the disease was being spread widely through infected needles used by drug addicts, as well as through homosexual intercourse. Walls began to go up in the mind. PWAs were seen as poor addicts, usually African-American. The particularly cautious used the connection between AIDS and drugs as a reason for legalizing drugs—needles would be cleaner.

Even when AIDS babies began filling special wards in city hospitals, even when it was discovered that the blood-donor pipeline had been contaminated, most Americans felt safe behind their walls. The realization began to take hold that heterosexual transmission of AIDS was not only a possibility, but already existed in our communities even as the scientific community argued about the extent of the danger of heterosexual transmission in the United States. The ugliness that has surrounded AIDS work has slowed and snarled the pace, but there is a living testimony among those who work with persons with AIDS and their survivors that they will be damned rather than give up work against AIDS.

FEARS AND STIGMA

Even though well-controlled studies repeatedly disprove any assertion that AIDS can be contracted through casual social contact, widespread fears continue. The long latency between viral exposure and any disease onset and the fact that most HIV carriers appear healthy further contribute to the uniqueness of the disease. AIDS elicits stigmatizing and prejudicial attitudes with respect to the perceived life-styles of PWAs because of its association with homosexuality, drug use and sexual behavior. Admittedly, most persons with AIDS are identified with groups scorned by society, and a large proportion of these persons are people of color.

While a few people are willing to disclose the fact that they have AIDS, most are apprehensive about disclosure. The difficulty or ease with which people face the prospect of disclosure is influenced by their attitude toward AIDS, their personal relationships and other relationships such as those with professionals, family members and significant others. There is a parallel in that gay and bisexual men, under the duress of the stigma of AIDS, have grown more circumspect about revealing their sexual orientation due to attacks and hate campaigns directed toward them by reactionary groups (Batchelor 1984). Large-scale public opinion polls confirm that the prevalence of harsh, judgmental and fearful attitudes concerning persons with AIDS continues (Fischer 1986; Siegel 1986; Kagay 1991).

During the past several years, proposals have been made to tattoo or quarantine persons with AIDS and HIV infection. Children with AIDS have been kept from attending school, and persons with AIDS have been denied health care, housing and employment owing to unwarranted fears of casual transmission (Young 1986; Brown 1989; Matthews & Neslund 1987). This suggests that some of the stigma associated with AIDS reflects misinformation about how the disease is transmitted and disdain and prejudice toward those affected.

Fear of AIDS in the workplace has significant consequences. Many health care professionals constantly worry about AIDS, a state of mind that may influence the quality of their work and dampen their enthusiasm for their jobs (Clever & Omann 1988; Keller 1988; Ostrow & Gayle 1986; White 1988). In a study of physicians in California, 35% were reluctant to provide care to AIDS patients (Olszewski 1988). In another study, 74% of a sample of California dentists (Gerbert 1987) said that they would rather refer people with AIDS to other providers. Thus, providers may be avoiding people known to have AIDS or to be HIV-positive. In one study, more than 80% of nurses said they would hesitate to perform mouth-to-mouth resuscitation on AIDS patients for fear of contracting the disease (Blumfield et al. 1987). In a case report on nursing care for a pediatric AIDS patient, Krener (1987) documented the child's extreme sensitivity to caretaker behavior.

Several authors have commented on countertransference problems in working with persons with AIDS (Dunkel & Hatfield 1986; Stevens & Muskin 1987). To avoid contact with HIV-infected people, some health care professionals are considering other careers (Gerbert 1987). Fear has also led health professionals to call for widespread HIV testing (Sherer 1988; Carey 1988; Weiner 1988). Such testing is not supported by public health authorities (Koop 1987; Osborn 1989), because of the potentially devastating impact on patients if confidentiality is breached (Wood & Philipson 1987).

Fear of AIDS centers around questions of death, sex and stigma, and is well documented (Bayer 1989; Navarro 1991). The overriding challenge is to confront AIDS proactively and to minimize the threat to communities, persons with AIDS, their survivors and health providers—to make a commitment to respond by allocating resources and providing comprehensive training programs. The incalculable cost of human suffering to people with little hope of recovery and to their survivors is tremendous, and can be reduced by rationally confronting the issue of AIDS.

CURRENT CHALLENGES

Even with the current state of the art of medical research, there is little reason to believe the quest for an AIDS vaccine will soon be successful. Unfortunately, the gap between identifying the cause of AIDS and finding a way to prevent, eradicate or control it is a wide one. The most difficult challenge is to provide care and treatment with dignity and concern for the individual and loved ones during the course of the illness and throughout the mourning process. Also, efforts to limit the spread of AIDS through education need to be focused on everyone since we are all at risk.

AIDS statistics are broken down by risk factors concerned with sexual behavior or drug use. Although these statistics enable us to understand the epidemic's component parts and how to slow its spread, this fragmentation and abstraction of the reality of AIDS is hazardous. First, we can easily lose sight of the big picture of the epidemic in a specific time and place in history. Second, these huge numbers understate the reality of AIDS. Despite a common belief that the epidemic has crested, many more people are becoming newly infected. In epicenters like New York City and Newark, we will probably experience at least one new HIV infection for each AIDS death. Barring some medical miracle, the effect of this disease on our daily lives and social institutions will deepen over the next generation (Drucker 1991).

Changes in our ideological beliefs about sexual habits and needle exchange programs are imperative. Coming to terms with our reflexive response to the needs of poor, inner-city families can only restore our covenant of responsibility with these families.

The estimated annual cost of treating a person infected with HIV is $5,150; the estimated annual cost of treating a person with full-blown AIDS is $32,000; and the lifetime cost is $85,333. Financing programs to care for people with AIDS who are living longer, thanks to drugs like azidothymidine (AZT) and dideoxydidine (DDI), providing a range of services—housing, counseling for intravenous drug users and their partners, child care—and developing bereavement programs for survivors must be proposed and acted upon by state and federal legislatures. In the face of such social upheaval, these services can make a huge difference. Mental health professionals must be less sanguine in their approach to the disease and instead mobilize groups of recovering addicts and infected women to organize as gay males have done up to now.

Denying abortion services to women who are infected with the AIDS virus requires investigation and immediate sanctions to comply with the law barring discrimination against disabled people (Navarro, 1991). Compassion toward disenfranchised groups seems light years away, but we must ask ourselves how we are contributing to the decimation of a large percentage of African-American and Hispanic people.

The arithmetic of the disease dramatizes the need not only to focus on the prevention of AIDS but also to develop drugs to prevent the progression of the disease. Further, we must instill compassion toward people who are suffering from the illness as well as their surviving families and loved ones. The implications for future generations are profound, although yet to be examined in a systematic way. Understanding how families and significant others are coping, and exploring resources that are available and needed, demands further study. Investigation of family relationships, resources, financial and emotional costs over the life and death of the person with AIDS requires professional attention.

Susan Sontag (1989) writes that we all have "dual citizenship" in the "kingdom of the well and the kingdom of the sick." Eventually we all pick up that second passport. But we need not travel alone. We have learned great lessons from the gay community, which we now have to extend to all families as we enter the second decade of AIDS.

CHAPTER 3

Bereavement Responses of Survivors of Persons Who Died of AIDS

The death of a valued person precipitates a major life crisis for most individuals. In an article published posthumously, Toynbee (1976) asserts that death is a dyadic event in which there are always "two parties to the suffering that death inflicts; and in the apportionment of this suffering, the survivor takes the brunt" (332). Toynbee's observation, published over a decade ago, is supported by the experience of legions of bereaved persons who experience the death of a loved one from AIDS.

Bereavement issues differ for different populations, and we see some differences in the patterning depending on the type of loss experienced. The groups of bereaved AIDS survivors are a population that has not been studied extensively. Survivors of AIDS deaths experience prejudice, stigma, devastation of large numbers of relatively young people, confrontations with mortality and multiple losses on a large scale, all of which exacerbate the normative grieving process.

Grief has many facets, but an understanding of the process helps the practitioner to meet the individual needs of the survivor of a person who has died of AIDS. Although professionals in the field of death education and counselling agree that grieving is essential in adjusting to the loss of a loved one, there remain numerous questions and even disagreements about how best to facilitate successful grief work.

The theoretical constructs of this chapter guide our beginning understanding of responses that contribute to AIDS bereavement. Cowan & Murphy (1985) suggest that the following factors be considered to sensitize professionals to grief among AIDS survivors: (1) the mode of death; (2) multiple, simultaneous deaths in a family; (3) the appraisal of the death event, that is, devastating, threatening or challenging; (4) the relationship between the deceased and bereaved prior to death, that is, valued or ambivalent; (5) coping skills; and (6) perception of social support. Based on hundreds of hours spent by the authors with a community of bereaved individuals grieving the loss of a significant person to AIDS, these six factors seemed most appropriate to guide our discussion.

MODE OF DEATH

The death of a significant other is consistently viewed as the most aversive of stressful life events (Holmes & Rahe 1967; Sarason, Johnson & Siegel 1978). Weisman (1973) suggests that untimely death (unexpected, premature or violent) has more devastating effects on bereaved persons than does timely (expected, accepted) death (see Chapter 1).

AIDS survivors have family members who were socially considered invisible and stigmatized, and the majority die out of phase with the expected life cycle. Children die before parents, parents die leaving young children or several persons in the same family network die in the same time period.

For the male couple, the loss of a partner to AIDS elicits a particularly complex set of responses. The lover may become idealized after death, and feelings of guilt may be experienced by the survivor, especially if he chose not to stay with his partner throughout the process of dying (Gilbert 1988). Furthermore, there is the chance of infection. The survivor may have given the deceased the disease or may have been infected by the deceased.

When the deceased is an addict, the family may experience intense feelings of failure and a reawakening of the unresolved mourning issues connected with earlier losses. Walker (1987) discusses surviving addicted spouses with one or more children, who are mourning and also experiencing anger and helplessness regarding the likely death of other family members.

Death from AIDS often sharpens family battles, compounding the survivor's isolation. It is essential to learn from survivors where they entered the course of the deceased's life/illness, which helps to understand what reorganization has taken place. Whether long or short, an adjustment period follows death, which provides some beginning time to accept it. Bowen (1987) has hypothesized an "emotional shock wave" that follows the death of a significant family member. Driven by anxiety, it moves throughout the family system, having an impact on many persons in that system, even those who may have been relatively uninvolved with the deceased.

Anticipatory Mourning

Most practitioners agree that the survivors who rally around the person with AIDS prior to death experience some emotional healing. Families, lovers and friends have stated they felt comfortable and at peace if they had been available during the death process.

A brief grief reaction may exist when the anticipatory grief period was of sufficient duration to allow for a "working-through process." The person with AIDS may have lived as long as five years or more, or died within a month of the first major infection leading to diagnosis. In cases in which the AIDS death was slow, most survivors reported having had opportunities to experience the full impact of their anticipated loss of the loved one prior to death. During this period difficult feelings can be expressed about the secret relationships between families of origin, procreation and function.

A major issue for a gay partner is his relationship with his deceased lover's parents or siblings. In some cases, surviving lovers sever the tie to their partners and suffer extreme guilt and anger. Others experience a reentry into their lover's family of origin and full participation with the family prior to and after the death. Heterosexual couples with an infected member feel isolated because the support systems typical of the gay community are perceived as not being available to them. AIDS may symbolize actual or suspected sexual infidelity or promiscuity, deviant drug use or homosexuality, all of which stigmatize survivors.

Wives of bisexual husbands initially experience feelings of rage, shame, confusion and betrayal. Coming to terms with the sexual orientation of their husbands and its implications prior to death helps them to make decisions about their families' immediate future.

Children whose parents die of AIDS often feel bewildered by the surrounding secrecy and isolation prior to and after the death. In large families, separation from the parent by death is often made worse by separation from brothers and sisters due to custody arrangements. Grandmothers in many situations assume responsibility for their grandchildren. Many custodial parents are unsure as to whether to discuss the circumstances of the parent's death, and often experience a lack of support and express feelings of being "out of sync."

Parents of adult children who provided support to their homosexual sons prior to death feel less angry and are more likely to provide support to other parents through support groups. Parents whose sons or daughters were IV drug abusers or prostitutes feel relieved for their adult children but describe the loss of the eternal hopes and dreams that these children would somehow change their behavior.

Suicide Survivor's Grief

Although all survivors are likely to experience grief reactions to various degrees, death from AIDS by suicide confronts the violent, rejection of the self, additionally burdening the bereaved. Whether suicide has been preceded by threats or is totally without prior clues, it usually wreaks havoc among the survivors, who are always unprepared. Lehrman (1956) found that pathological grief reactions were more frequent when death was both sudden and unexpected. The age of the deceased may also influence the unexpectedness of the death.

Death by suicide was quite common in the IV drug use subculture prior to AIDS. Overdose deaths primarily come from taking a much stronger than usual dose of heroin, so that whatever tolerance has been developed is not sufficient to prevent a fatal respiratory depression (Corless & Lindeman 1988). Families and survivors of a loved one who has died by an overdose when diagnosed with AIDS state that it is a quick and euphoric release from a troubled life with the potential of dying from physical debilitation, pain and troubled interpersonal relationships. Some survivors have become involved in rescue attempts prior to the death and continue to experience anger and helplessness regarding the likely death of other family members.

Out of intense feelings of love and grief after the death of a gay partner with AIDS, thoughts of suicide are not unusual. A study by Marzuk et al. (1988) demonstrated a substantially increased risk for suicide among males with AIDS. It was found that in 1985 in New York City, the risk of suicide in men aged twenty to fifty-nine who were diagnosed with AIDS was thirty-six times that of men the same age without the diagnosis, and sixty-six times that of the general population.

Psychological stressors related to withdrawal of family support, loss of friends or lovers (often to AIDS), the social stigma and the unwillingness to endure a protracted, painful illness serve as precipitating factors in the suicide of persons with AIDS. Survivors often understand the reason for suicide, unlike the general population of suicide survivors, hope that the reason will assuage their guilt.

The impact of suicide by persons with AIDS on survivors reflects the cumulative sense of suffering pain, being a burden to others, and experiencing the shame that society heaps upon both the homosexual person and the intravenous drug user. Repeated hospitalizations, multiple treatment regimens and the consequences of a dementia that will worsen all contribute to questions about life and death for the PWA. Some survivors who are confronted with these multiple stressors are more likely to develop physical and psychological disorders than those who are experiencing stress from a single source (Brown & Harris 1978).

In certain cases, survivors have participated in and facilitated the "rational suicide" of their loved one with AIDS. They have taken their cues from the dying person or felt that suicide was a better choice. The survivor counseled and encouraged personal growth and a dignified end to a pointless death in the face of dementia or coma. With such a future, those who had enjoyed higher self-esteem, but lacked the adaptation gained from earlier suffering, were given the permission and assistance to die without guilt. Some lovers of gay men acknowledge feeling empowered in assisting their loved ones to die, and are consoled in knowing they are at peace.

Families, too, feel consoled by the thought that their adult children saw no other viable alternative, and that when compared to dementia or great pain, suicide was an appropriate choice. Some other surviving family members feel that they would be more at peace and less guilty if their son had persevered in giving to and receiving from others the growth and love still available in the unfinished business of life (Corless & Lindeman 1988).

MULTIPLE DEATHS

Eliot (1972) estimates that there have been some 100 million man-made deaths (e.g., automobile accidents, shootings and terrorist activities) in the twentieth century. Admittedly, man-made death has tended to replace epidemics as the cause of megadeath. Death from AIDS has not yet matched the carnage of the series of wars the United States has fought since World War I, but the extent of its impact is far from over. Not only are we encountering a high proportion of young people dying, but five, six or seven members of one family are dying within a short period of time (Walker 1987).

We are just now beginning to confront the bleak realities of numerous family members dying of AIDS, and of the large community of mourners. Children, the sexual partners and friends, parents and lovers of gay men, health care professionals, are all coping with multiple losses. The psychosocial implications are anguishing.

Most young mothers suffering from AIDS and their families are poor and African-American or Hispanic. They often live in inadequate housing, have had poor access to health care, and rely on marginal and stressed social supports from persons who are also confronted with repeated losses. These mothers are experiencing their own illness, as well as that of their infants. There are hundreds of cases of infants who, after their mother's death, are virtually abandoned and receive care from either hospital staff or the foster care system. Children who do go home from the hospital often live with mothers and siblings who are dying or have lost a father to AIDS. The illness and death of the child is directly related to the mother's transmission of the disease. This dynamic adds to the horror of coping with the illness and the anticipated death of one's child (Foster 1988).

The pain and grief attached to the death of a child always remains and, since unresolved, can affect other siblings. To complete her accommodation to her lingering sorrow and develop a better self-image, the mother must build a coherent bridge between her past and her present. If her rage, bitterness and guilt are to be resolved, she needs to examine honestly, and without accusation of herself or others, just what her circumstances were at the time she was infected with AIDS. Some mothers (particularly those who have been addicted in the past) report that they resort to drugs or alcohol to hide from their feelings of guilt and loss.

The heavy emotional scars experienced by children whose parents, siblings, aunts, uncles or friends have died from the disease are overwhelming.

Most children cannot find the words to express the grief and pain they are feeling. They expend a great deal of energy trying to keep their feelings buried since the environment, hardened with stigma, does not facilitate free expression. But suppressing emotions does not eliminate the emotions. Rather, they manifest themselves in many ways—guilt, anger, tension and uneasiness around other children. The numbing aroused by the disbelief and efforts to keep the secret limit their responsiveness.

Many situations have been reported where the parents have been summoned to a major city to learn that their son is dying of AIDS, while simultaneously coping with the secret of his homosexual life and the pending death of his partner. For the parents, the son and the partner, there are disturbing feelings that need resolution to aid in the mourning. Trauma is paramount when a wife has contracted AIDS from her bisexual husband and she is mourning his death, anticipating her own death and leaving her children fighting the infections she is experiencing, and also preparing custody rights.

Martin (1989) and Martin et al. (1988, 1989) indicate the presence of growing numbers of gay men who exhibit signs of post-traumatic stress disorder (PTSD), which they describe as characterized by symptom development following a distressing event or events outside the range of usual human experience, such as multiple and continuing deaths in one's immediate surroundings. Symptoms include intrusive and avoidant thoughts and emotions about AIDS. Martin et al. (1989) report that the annual incidence of AIDS-related bereavement went from 2% in 1981, to 18% in 1985, to 23% in 1987, with one-third of the study participants having lost one or more close friends within the same year. As incidents of AIDS-related bereavement rise and more men experience multiple losses, Martin et al. (1989) predict a rise in symptoms of PTSD, demoralization and illicit drug use.

Erich Lindemann (1944) states: "One of the big obstacles to grief work seem to be the fact that many people try to avoid both the intense distress connected with the grief experience and necessary expression of emotion. . . . They required considerable persuasion to yield to the grief process, which would enable them to accept the discomfort of bereavement" (7). If the survivor does not accept the pain of loss, subsequent grief work cannot proceed. The clinician must continuously persuade the survivor to accept the grief rather than flee from the painful feelings via medication, substance abuse and distracting behaviors. This process is very difficult for survivors of AIDS deaths who have experienced bereavement overload through a series of deaths.

Hirsch and Enlow (1984) say that "bereavement overload" occurs when an individual has not completed the bereavement process for one person when another dies. The pervasive, unrelenting feelings of sorrow, loss and abandonment are overwhelming. The magnitude of the loss must be validated before survivors experiencing multiple losses can think about their feelings of abandonment, fear and anger. This area of multiple loss has been greatly neglected. It is common for survivors, especially those living in AIDS epicenters, to endure multiple bereavements due to the deaths of persons from AIDS while, at the same time, some are facing the possibility of their own death.

APPRAISAL OF THE DEATH EVENT

Hyman and Woog (1982) report that it is the client's perception of the event as stress-producing that is crucial to treatment rather than the event itself. This is an important factor when working with a diversity of survivors with different special characteristics in lifestyles and relationships, including gay men, bisexual men and women, IV drug users, drug and alcohol abusers, heterosexual women, adolescents, elders, lesbians, hemophiliacs and blood product recipients, people of color, people who are poor, the sexual partners of any of the above and infants or children.

Following an upsetting event, individuals cognitively appraise the situation to determine personal demands, constraints and available resources. Hartsough (1985) differentiates agent (AIDS) produced stress (e.g., death of family members) from response (official and social agency) produced stress (e.g., interviews by social workers or coroner's office), and notes that both are potential sources of stress for survivors.

Understanding the perception of death from AIDS requires understanding the phenomenon of widespread, intensely negative reactions to persons with AIDS. These negative reactions shape the behavior of survivors and limit the effectiveness of grief work. Many families are hurt and feel victimized. Victimization is defined here as "the overpowering of an individual or a family with physical or psychological trauma, resulting in feelings of helplessness, shame, and distrust" (Boss 1988, 4).

In family victimization, the loss is not only the death of a loved one but also a loss of family pride and confidence. The family feels shame. Fossum and Mason (1986), using a family systems perspective, discuss shame, and suggest that it is a family phenomenon. Entire families can be immobilized by their loss of pride, especially when something happens that is stigmatizing. In the pandemic of AIDS, families not only have to deal with the trauma of the illness and the death of a loved one but also must bear the burden of societal hostility at a time when they are most in need of social support.

The person bereaved from a loved one's death from AIDS sustains a double loss, one of the person and the other of the opportunity to publicly mourn the loss. This occurs for two reasons: the death was not socially sanctioned, or there are controversies and stigma related to a specific type of loss. Since a person who dies from AIDS is not valued by society, there is a lack of needed social support for the survivor to face the pain. If the relationship has not been openly acknowledged, often there are no bereavement rituals to help one cope with the loss.

In an effort to gain some control and understanding over what appears to be a meaningless, unmanageable event, the bereaved often engage in an obsessional review of the circumstances of the death. They may wonder how, in what should be a fair and just world, this could be happening to them. They feel shame since the death is stigmatized, and they may not see a clear course of action in the face of such loss.

Our dominant myths reflect our dominant values. Many myths about the death of a family member exist in Western society. Our culture warns us against "wallowing in pity" or "feeling sorry for ourselves" and describes the expression of loss and sorrow in negative terms: breaking down, falling apart, getting hysterical, acting like a baby. This negative influence supports the bereaved person's wish to avoid the pain that follows discussion of feelings. Thus feelings are unexpressed and mourning is often delayed.

An additional difficulty for the survivor is that there are no models or culturally prescribed roles for AIDS mourners in our society. This makes it difficult for the bereaved person to know how to act or feel. With the absence of such guidelines, there is an increase of ambiguity. The most pernicious aspect of survivorship is the accompanying ambiguity as survivors face the unpredictable. The uncertainty and ambiguity of such situations make it difficult for the survivor to take precautions against harm (for example losing valuable possessions previously shared with the deceased), fostering stress in a situation that is already overburdened.

Some survivors may be relieved when a death finally occurs, especially when the deceased has been suffering or the survivor has been the caretaker during a long, drawn-out illness. This response is not a statement about the feelings or lack of feeling for the deceased, but more a reflection of the griever's response to the alleviation of suffering and the termination of responsibilities. Survivors also may feel relief simply because they themselves are not dying or because their relationship with the deceased was marked by a great deal of conflict or oppression (Rando 1985).

Societal myths as well as AIDS-related stigma and shame discredit the survivors. Goffman (1963) states that the focus of social psychological research on stigma is not on the mark itself as much as on the social relationships in which a particular mark is defined as shameful or discrediting. The authors are concerned with the social psychological processes through which people are discredited when they are perceived to be associated with AIDS.

Like other life-threatening illnesses, AIDS confronts even the noninfected with the reality of death, provoking what Schultz (1962) describes as the "fundamental anxiety." When people interact with AIDS survivors, hear AIDS discussed or simply read about it in a newspaper, they are reminded of their own mortality; their day-to-day sense of reality is challenged in a profoundly disturbing way. According to Schultz, the pragmatic objective of daily life (the "natural attitude") is to construct experiences that avoid this fundamental anxiety.

Because of its prevalence among already stigmatized groups, persons with AIDS and their loved ones can easily be exploited for ideological and political purposes. A Houston mayoral candidate (and former mayor), for example, publicly joked that his solution to the city's AIDS problem would be to "shoot the queers" (Shilts 1987). Such a political use of AIDS heightens the stigma associated with the disease and affects survivors negatively.

Similarly, persons who did not contract AIDS through homosexual behavior or drug use have often been categorized as "innocent victims" (Albert 1986), as have their families. For example, a *Newsweek* caption early in the epidemic described a teenage hemophiliac and an infant with AIDS as "the most blameless victims," conveying pity for them and for their survivors. The opposite, of course, is a blameable victim, that is one who was infected with HIV through homosexual behavior or drug use. Survivors of such persons are, by association, blameworthy.

The societal perception of AIDS survivors is complicated by the epidemic's association with already marginalized groups. Consequently, most individuals do not respond to survivors experiencing a loss, but respond to them as mourning a gay man, IV drug abuser or minority person who died from a lethal and transmissible disease (Herek & Glunt 1988). Because of the dialectical relation between cultural ideologies and individual attitudes, any attempt to eradicate AIDS-related stigma for survivors must focus on public policy strategies to establish clear social norms of respect and compassion for persons with AIDS and their survivors.

RELATIONSHIP BETWEEN DECEASED AND BEREAVED

Death from AIDS results in survivors facing normal life transitions (loss of spouse, lover, child or of peers) at a much earlier stage of the life cycle than developmentally appropriate. The relative young age at death of most persons is a factor with which survivors contend. Cohen and Willisch (1978) suggest key factors determining how families will respond during bereavement: (1) the family's stage in the life cycle; (2) the maturational and chronological age of the individuals involved; (3) the quality of constraints that are unique to the particular family; and (4) how flexible the family has been in earlier times.

AIDS affects and is affected by the responses of important others in the bereaved person's environment. How do families interact with their loved ones, once AIDS is detected, and then, when the person dies? Does AIDS change relationships? How do families disclose the death to extended family and friends? Our interviews with survivors led to the realization that it is neither possible nor desirable to oversimplify complex relationships, and that our examinations have to be both systematic and individualized. The following discussion will provide some insight into what survivors experience in their relationships prior to the death of a loved one.

Because AIDS is transmitted largely through behaviors associated with homosexuality and/or intravenous drug use, it is socially unspeakable. Consequently, family members hold back thoughts, emotions and feelings from virtually everyone, even clergy and professional counselors. In some families, AIDS, homosexuality or IV drug use are taboo topics of conversation, not only between the immediate family and others, but also within the family. This deadly silence compounds the emotional devastation that families undergo during the bereavement process.

The tendency toward blaming and judging in American society is seen as a critical barrier in some family relationships. Blaming stands where action, assistance and acceptance of reality should stand and has interfered with the functions of a number of families who have seen their relatives as untouchable, evil and deserving of their illness.

The closeness of the relationship between the mourner and the deceased is directly related to the intensity of the grief reaction (Bugen 1977). If the relationship to the deceased is seen as central, the grief reaction will be intense. If the relationship is considered peripheral, the grief reaction will be mild. The grief reaction is likely to be more intense when the survivor is infected. Any one or some combination of the following criteria may define a central relationship between a survivor and a loved one.

First, the most powerful of all bereaved conditions, and the most likely to sustain a sense of hopelessness is when the deceased person's presence was so profound that there is no life without them. The survivor typically feels as though life is meaningless or senseless without the loved one. Expressions such as "What am I going to do now?" or "I wish I were dead, too" are very common. Age offers little protection from these feelings.

Second, for the deceased to be considered central, it is not enough for the mourner merely to have loved the deceased. Survivors must see the nurturance and love of the person who has died as having been a vital source of daily support—a mother's reassuring smile, a partner's warm embrace, a child's delight in winning a game—the loss of which is felt deeply and constantly.

Centrality may also refer to a person to whom the survivor had become behaviorally committed through daily activity. The most obvious examples are the death of an adult child or lover for whom a mother or lover assumed daily caregiving responsibilities, such as bathing, making breakfast and helping to soothe physical and emotional pain. Even a cantankerous gay person may be sorely missed by a "buddy" who daily delivered meals, providing one of the more vital moments in the buddy's day.

Lastly, a central relationship may be with a person whose very existence serves as a reminder and symbol for our hopes and beliefs. Thousands of individuals mourned the death from AIDS of Liberace and Rock Hudson.

Most of these mourners had never met either performer, but experienced their deaths as a loss.

On the other side of this pendulum are the minimally important relationships referred to as peripheral (Bugen 1977). A peripheral relationship refers to a person whose presence is both felt and respected but whose loss is not viewed or experienced as irreplaceable. Relationships with a neighbor, a co-worker, a distant family member, teachers or hospital personnel, in which the survivor had recognized the contributions of the deceased (both positive and negative) but had not extended the relationship, may be considered peripheral.

COPING SKILLS

According to Bandura (1977), self-efficacy involves judgments about how well one can organize and carry out courses of behavior necessary to cope with prospective situations involving ambiguous, unpredictable and stressful elements in the environment. Whether a survivor engages in trying to cope, and how long she/he will persist in coping, depends on the belief or expectation at the outset.

The particular sources of stress that characterize a survivor's coping in the AIDS epidemic include a high AIDS mortality rate, the youthfulness of persons with AIDS at death, the concerns with transmission, the capacity of AIDS to debilitate and disfigure, the major life-style changes required by the illness, the impact of AIDS on relationships, the uncertainty and fear AIDS engenders in others, the stigma attached to and internalized by the person with AIDS and significant others and the inaccessibility of sources of comfort and support (Wong, Allen & Moore 1988; King 1989; Flaskerud 1987; Dane 1989; Christ & Wiener 1985).

The bereaved may have unexplainable somatic symptoms or changes in personality that mimic those of the deceased. For example, a surviving gay lover experienced recurrent night sweats similar to his lover, but when tested was negative. Bowlby (1973) points out that anger and weeping are necessary, biologically ingrained responses leading toward the recognition that the loss is final. The inability to cry or rage at the loss frequently stems from the bereaved trying not to "fall apart."

Guilt and shame are often reported by AIDS survivors (Christ & Wiener 1985; Dane 1989; Lomax & Sandler 1988). The concept of survivor guilt was first introduced into contemporary psychiatric literature by Niederland (1981), who described a severe and persevering guilt complex affecting survivors of the Holocaust. After a symptom-free interval, survivors developed symptoms such as depression, anhedonia, anxiety, hyperamnesia and psychosomatic conditions.

Niederland believed that these symptoms were identifications with loved ones who had not survived and ascribed to them a deep and pervasive sense of guilt. He further believed that the survivors' prior ambivalent attitudes toward, for example, a deceased parent, and the rage a youngster experienced toward the parent, were important factors and should be recognized in the treatment of survivors. Chodoff (1985) emphasizes the survivors' need to suffer and to memorialize their generation. Danieli (1985) proposes that guilt is an unconscious attempt to deny or undo the experience of passive helplessness that many AIDS survivors undergo.

Modell (1971) broadens the concept of survivor guilt. He states that survivor guilt stems from a biologically based concern for and sensitivity to the pain of significant others, making it difficult to be comfortable if they are not. Survivor guilt occurs in two forms, one of which is separation guilt, the belief on the part of the child that growing up and separating from the mother will damage and even destroy her. The other form of survivor guilt is guilt based upon the belief that death is at someone's else's expense. It was reported to the authors that survivor guilt was expressed by a number of adolescents in a therapy group for AIDS survivors. They wished that they had died rather than their idealized mothers. The tragic death of the teenagers' mothers provoked a rekindling of earlier separation and guilt issues.

Another example reported was of an older mother whose daughter, an IV drug user, died of AIDS. In comparing her life with that of her daughter's, she felt her own life to be less worthy. Her low self-esteem and guilt about surviving prompted her comments about the wish to exchange places so that she had died and her daughter had been saved.

Much of the normal ambivalence in human relationships is denied or repressed by survivors. For example, when a homosexual adolescent dies, many parents feel guilty about anger they expressed regarding their child's life-style. Suddenly, these remembered outbursts seem ominous, threatening and hostile, and thoughts about them promote excessive guilt, which is difficult to express. Some parents find it easier to deny that such thoughts or feelings ever existed.

Bereaved mothers who were the chief caretakers during lengthy illnesses of their adult homosexual sons often repress the hostile feelings that they experienced when their sons were angry, uncommunicative or seemingly unappreciative of their mother's acceptance of their illness and their lover. During a group meeting, these mothers told the authors that their son's death awakened the pain of their earlier loss in learning that their son was gay. These feelings were troubling and conflicted, and never completely resolved.

While anger is a typical response of any bereaved person, for AIDS survivors the anger is exacerbated by some of the specific social characteristics of the epidemic. Newmark (1984) writes about the anger the person and significant others feel at being treated like social pariahs. Morin, Charles & Malyon (1984) indicate that anger is often expressed in political form, focusing on government inaction in research on and treatment of AIDS, or on mistreatment of people with AIDS and their survivors.

Another mother could not understand or accept the personality changes that are common during AIDS dementia. She found it difficult to express her hostility toward her son, and blamed the visiting nurse for administering the wrong medication. Misdirected anger and ambivalence toward the deceased are normal ways of coping. The loss of a daughter or son to AIDS entails anger, dashed hopes and the interruption of shared plans. Anger at the deceased for having deserted the bereaved is perplexing to those who will acknowledge only positive feelings toward the loved person.

Children often experience murderous wishes during the lengthy illness of a sibling or parent. After the death, the child suppresses these wishes and fears that the wishes magically caused the death. Another form of guilt that older children find difficult to verbalize concerns their negative responses to the devastating effects the disease had on the physical appearance of their parent(s). Withdrawal from the parent promoted feelings of guilt, which was experienced as self-loathing after the death.

It is crucial that clinicians understand the dynamics that are involved in these situations so that they can work with the hidden guilt and anger. Helping survivors cope with and control anxiety, maintain hope and avoid becoming psychologically dysfunctional are important tasks. Universalization and verbalization help survivors forgive themselves for their human response to the devastating effects of AIDS.

PERCEPTIONS OF SOCIAL SUPPORT

Although we know that the main source of support for survivors in the aftermath of a loved one's death must come from within the person, this internal strength is initially weak and takes some time to develop. In the immediate aftermath of the death there is always confusion, disorganization, anger, resentment, despair and sometimes relief, all of which take their toll in terms of even the strongest individual's ability to respond rationally and effectively. Often there is a great gap between the survivor's ability to develop the internal resources necessary to deal with the death and the swift emotional impact the loss generates. The result is that the person is left floating in a limbo of grief so severe that the capacity for survival, let alone substantive functioning, is impaired. It is at this point that support systems can serve as sources of practical and emotional support for the survivor experiencing a transition.

In the last twenty years, social scientists have focused a great deal of attention on the role played by social supports in preventing disease, maintaining health and alleviating or buffering the impact of illness and death on the patient and those close to her/him (Adelman 1989; Bloom 1982; Zich & Temoshok 1987).

Caplan and Killilea (1976) define a support system as "an enduring pattern of continuous or intermittent ties that play a significant part in maintaining the psychological and physical integrity of the individual over time" (41). Social support is defined from a communication perspective by Albrecht and Adelman (1987), who see it as observable patterns of communication that reduce uncertainty about the situation, the self, the other or the relationship, enhancing a perception of control over one's life. A support network is defined by Walker, MacBride and Vachon (1977) as "that set of personal contacts through which the individual maintains her social identity and receives emotional support, material aid and services, and new social contacts" (35).

In addition to types of support, Zich and Temoshok (1987) indicate that current, more sophisticated research also approaches social supports in terms of perceived availability of support, perceived desirability of support, frequency of use and perceived helpfulness, harmfulness or satisfaction with the support. Pilisuk and Minkler (1985) and Zich and Temoshok (1987) note that the effectiveness of micro level support systems is dependent on the adequacy of macro level programs and policies, from which they derive access to basic necessities such as income maintenance, housing and other services.

It has been suggested that there are two AIDS epidemics—an epidemic of HIV infection and an epidemic of fear. The level and intensity of fear about AIDS have been apparent in the vehement reactions of many people when they have learned that a close family member or friend has died from AIDS. The "silent treatment" is probably the most oppressive and least recognized form of emotional abuse. Nothing one can say or do can bring it to an end. Belittling the survivor, either publicly or privately, is also likely to be devastating. This form of abuse is particularly vicious because the survivor is doomed to lose. Some react to the survivor's plight by minimizing the problem and disparaging the feelings the survivor may be experiencing. The survivor fears acting in self-defense, doubts her/himself, and begins to self-blame for being attached to the deceased.

As with the initial diagnosis of AIDS, the time of death invariably stresses the family system. The greatest source of the survivor's difficulty is the secret with which they lived. Fears of loss of confidentiality, stigmatization, isolation, loss of housing, termination from employment and abandonment by family, friends, neighbors and co-workers are not unfounded. The need for support is great.

Children have been isolated in schools when an immediate family member has died of AIDS. Many gay men have kept their partner's death a secret at the workplace, taking personal time rather than time specifically allocated for mourning their partner's death. In addition to the actual loss of a lover, these men experience a subtle but more corrosive loss when their self-esteem is damaged by social attitudes that deny the legitimacy of their grief. By withholding from them the right or the time to grieve, society only adds to their sense of guilt and worthlessness. In the first stage of mourning, these grieving men are unable to evaluate the appropriateness of other people's expectations of them. Some remain numb and isolated, and make every effort not to violate society's taboos by reminding others or themselves of their very real dilemmas. Instead they use their energy to repress or deny their feelings. They cannot yet cope with them effectively and therefore refuse to face the fact that their lives have changed irrevocably.

Some survivors are HIV-infected, and heightened and sustained stress may be associated with immunosuppression (Kielcolt-Glaser & Glaser 1987). Stress reduction techniques, and social support, may enhance immune functioning. Coates et al. (1987) suggest that the AIDS virus may be temporarily "held in check" through psychosocial factors.

Even when family and friends remain available and supportive, efforts to help the bereaved person to avoid grief may not be helpful. It is only when survivors can at last acknowledge pain, doubts and fears, when they no longer feel it necessary to present a false picture to themselves and others of how splendidly they are coping that the transition to life can happen without the deceased.

Talking with other survivors whose loved one died from AIDS can reassure a person that she/he is not going crazy and that it is acceptable to feel certain pain and relief. Although everyone who has a serious problem generally finds that only another person with the same problem truly understands all its complexities, getting together with other survivors who have had the same experience is particularly important. This is helpful because of the secrecy, shame and guilt that have characterized the AIDS environment.

Adelman (1989) states that few empirical studies have addressed the social support needs of AIDS survivors because of the highly sensitive and stigmatizing ramifications of AIDS and the historic distrust of many gay men and minorities for social science research. However, some empirical studies, clinical observations and personal accounts provide insight into a variety of aspects of the role social supports play in coping with AIDS.

For gay men, Fischer (1988) finds that the more comfortable gay men are with being gay, the greater their involvement with gay social networks to help them cope with their lover's deaths. The above reasoning is also consistent with research on help-seeking that suggests that acceptance of one's condition is an important determinant of seeking help or support. Until this occurs, support-seeking is highly self-threatening, and may be avoided. This would imply that gay men who are uncomfortable with being gay would be less apt to seek help to cope with their lover's death than those who are more comfortable. Unknowingly, societal values in response to the AIDS epidemic may be moving toward making gay men less, rather than more, comfortable with their sexual orientation. If gay men become fearful of prejudice and discrimination, this may lead to the rejection of gay networks for support, especially by individuals who are ambivalent about their homosexuality.

Wolcott et al. (1986) assessed fifty homosexual and bisexual men on a number of issues, including social supports. They report finding moderately small current social networks, and say that 52% of the respondents reported one or fewer family members in their current social network. The authors attribute this to the high level of estrangement between gay men and their families.

Adelman (1989) looks at the application to persons with AIDS of Taylor's (1983–84) theory of cognitive adaptation to threatening events, which includes: search for meaning to try to understand and explain why the crisis happened; work to restore self-esteem; and trying to gain a sense of control over life events. Adelman maintains that this theory is useful for organizing the existential, personal and pragmatic concerns of persons with AIDS and for understanding the function of social supports.

Social support is not always positive (Adelman 1989). For example, very dense social networks may prevent someone from seeking needed professional help, or support may counter the person's perception of independence, autonomy and privacy, and thus undermine the experience of personal control. Emotional support may be difficult to give and get if the survivor is in the process of coping with death in a way that is different from the mourning experiences of her/his primary supporters.

Overall, informal support networks reduce the need for professional help and can buffer the impact of the loss and aid in coping with life crises. Adelman (1989) emphasizes the importance of community support systems to prevent a drain on the primary support system. She says that "serious, chronic illness (death) places unrealistic demands on supporters, depleting personal resources such as time, physical and mental energy, and finances. Burnout is not uncommon" (36).

In articles concerned with gay relationships, Lovejoy (1989) and Adelman (1989) refer to the development of a "we" by the commingling of identities as part of the couple's relational definition. These authors are among the first who directly address the impact of AIDS on the gay male couple relationship. The surviving lover must reconstruct his own identity after his partner's death. Death means that surviving partners must rebuild their concepts of self, and must manage daily lives that are no longer predicated on merged identities. The shift from complete immersion in taking care of the lover to the isolation that follows his death creates disjunctive role changes. The need for social support is paramount in long-term gay relationships (Lovejoy 1989). In addition, Marzuk et al. (1988) note that during the bereavement period there is a propensity toward suicide for lovers of people who have died of AIDS, further underscoring the need for social supports.

The role and nature of friendships as social supports has received little attention in the literature. Lovejoy (1989) states that gay friendship networks, which can be very close and sustaining, are at times acknowledged, but are often referred to as "gay families" or "homosexual families." This imprecise use of the word family suggests that these friendship networks have something in common with families in terms of how they function or what they provide. Calling them families obscures that they are friendships, emotional bonding without any legal or biological ties. Friends are the main source of emotional and practical support for gay survivors, although some feel "let down" by friends.

Families are or are assumed to be a major source of social support for the bereaved. For homosexual men and IV drug abusers, however, this cannot be assumed. Often gay men and IV drug abusers are estranged from their families. Some gay men have unique and uneven patterns of family relationships, and receive a great deal of support from other gay friends. This is not the case in the drug abuser's community.

MENTAL HEALTH PROFESSIONALS

Public attitudes toward AIDS survivors have an impact on their social, emotional and physical experience after the death of a loved one. The process of asking professionals to understand extremely complex issues is difficult.

A high level of psychological distress among professionals working with people with AIDS is reported in the literature (Lopez & Getzel 1987; Treiber, Shaw & Malcolm 1987), and even hospital workers who have little contact with AIDS patients report high stress related to this contact (Pleck et al. 1988). Although these stresses are generally based on unfounded fears of transmission, the stress is conveyed to the bereaved survivors.

Kelly, et al. (1987a, 1987b), Merrill, Laux and Thornby (1989) and Royse and Birge (1987) all report that both physicians and medical students are susceptible to or already have significantly negative and stigmatizing attitudes toward persons with AIDS and their survivors. These attitudes translate into less empathy. Doctors, nurses and other hospital staff are also reported by Douglas, Kalman and Kalman (1985) and Wallack (1989) to have significantly homophobic attitudes and negative attitudes toward AIDS. They indicate that the quality of care received by people with AIDS is seriously impaired by homophobia and fear of AIDS.

Eliminating AIDS-related stigma requires massive education among health care and mental health professionals. AIDS-related stigma is a problem for all of society. It imposes severe hardships on the people who are its targets, and it ultimately interferes with treating this massive community of bereaved AIDS survivors. Creating a social climate conducive to a rational, effective and compassionate response to this epidemic will be a start toward tolerating differences and dissipating the prejudice that is a major obstacle to grief resolution.

IMPLICATIONS FOR PRACTITIONERS

Bereaved survivors who have experienced the loss of a loved one from AIDS do not always perceive mental health professionals as helpful. Murphy (1986) reported his findings from a study of people who survived a disaster.

They indicated that professionals lacked understanding of their need to repeat verbally their perceptions and their frequent feelings of self-blame.

Since clinicians are often in a position to intervene with survivors, it is important they be aware of the climate of stigma and discrimination as well as the stages and symptoms of grief. Assessment based on the nature, duration and expression of mourning, and the survivor's cultural and ethnic beliefs, can influence the practitioners' interventions. Outreach to survivors of AIDS deaths is essential. Often the survivors have experienced the callousness and fears of professionals and have been labeled "resistant." Instead of understanding their way of coping and their expression of stoicism as an adaptive strategy to protect themselves from further pain in an already taboo area, unsubstantiated assumptions have been made about this bereaved population.

Some survivors may seek help, and the practitioner must seize the opportunity that the crisis of loss offers. Crisis is both an opportunity and a danger. Knowledge of crisis intervention and empathy regarding issues of isolation and symptomatology of grief are essential.

Survivors of people who have died from AIDS constitute a relatively new population of grievers for whom there are few guidelines for care and few resources to consult. Interventions must take into account the present unspeakable nature of death by AIDS. This can have a profound effect on the grief resolution of all survivors.

CHAPTER 4

Intervening with Children and Adolescents

In this second decade of AIDS, it is projected that about 10 million children and adolescents will become orphans (*New York Times*, 1991). Worldwide attention and publicity focused on the AIDS epidemic has essentially by-passed bereaved children whose parents have died from AIDS.

The death of a parent from AIDS is one of the most emotionally stressful events that can happen to a child. The parent-child relationship is viewed as the crucible for personality development (Bowlby 1969; Mahler, Pine & Bergman 1975; Winnicott 1971). The loss of such a relationship has major implications for healthy adaptation (Bowlby 1980a).

Some have observed that a parent's death during childhood is a psychic trauma. Krueger (1983) states that "the real rather than the symbolic or fantasized loss of a parent during development imposes an actual trauma, with implications for intrapsychic organization during development" (582). Worden (1982) also supports the theory that the loss of a parent through death is a trauma. Black (1978), in her review of the literature on the bereaved child, concludes that a parent's death usually constitutes a massive psychic trauma because an immature ego cannot sustain the grief process without suffering injury. Not only is the death of a parent a debilitating experience for children and adolescents to endure, but equally traumatic is learning of the parent's diagnosis of a fatal and stigmatizing illness—AIDS.

Children and adolescents who are survivors of a parental death from AIDS experience both trauma and grief. A disproportionate percentage of bereaved children in families where one or both parents have died from AIDS come from African-American and Hispanic families, and some of these children also have a diagnosis of AIDS or are HIV-positive. The majority of mothers in these families and/or their partners were drug abusers, living in urban areas and suffering from poverty and discrimination. Other mothers, having acquired HIV from heterosexual transmission rather than their own drug use, made the often shocking discovery of their infection after their child tested HIV-positive or was diagnosed with AIDS. The noninfected children or adolescents in these families experience multiple deaths.

Although death impacts the individual throughout the life cycle, in this chapter we will discuss latency and adolescent children. Clinical interventions with these diverse populations will be reflected through case illustrations. Guidelines will be offered to professionals assisting children and adolescents to explore the traumatic factors of AIDS that influence the bereavement process.

CONCEPTUAL UNDERPINNINGS

Because of their vulnerability, children and adolescents who lose a family member to AIDS face unique issues as they grieve. Children and adolescents in families affected by HIV often have watched their families disintegrate before their eyes. They struggle to make sense of a senseless situation and to feel in control, even as they confront circumstances over which they ultimately have no control. In addition to parental loss, many children and adolescents experience the death of a sibling or close relative.

A prominent theme or consistent question of professionals has to do with the child's capacity to mourn in the face of parental loss. In recent years, we have come to understand that children are capable of a wide range of grief responses. Their expression of grief is influenced by their level of development, their personality and their cultural milieu. The general literature on child and adolescent bereavement is applicable to the population of survivors whose parent(s) died from AIDS.

In Freud's (1917) classic exposition of grief work in "Mourning and Melancholia," and throughout the bereavement literature, the ability to express grief and sorrow following the death of a loved one has been associated with coping and adaptation. With children, however, the situation is not always so clear. Bowlby (1961) states that infants as young as six months old experience mourning reactions identical to those observed in adults. Wolfenstein (1966), in contrast, views adolescence as the time when individuals acquire the capacity to mourn.

In between these polar positions are those who believe the ability to grieve is acquired during childhood, as ego functions mature and the ability to comprehend the finality of death is achieved. Anna Freud (1960) specifies that, in order for mourning to be possible, an individual must possess certain ego capacities, among them reality testing, acceptance of the reality principle and control of id tendencies. These capacities are assumed to be absent in the very young child.

Furman (1974) confirms the usefulness of psychological assistance to the bereaved. He states that when a child's parent dies, the child faces an in-comparable stress that threatens further personality development. This out-come can be averted if the child (as young as a toddler) is helped to mourn the parent as fully as possible. Some clinicians assert that the negative impact of the loss of a parent in childhood on the personality of the child is un-avoidable. In their view, crisis intervention immediately after the event in no way diminishes the danger to the psychological health of the members of the bereaved family (Pollack et al. 1975). Osterweis, Solomon and Green (1984) conclude that early loss raises the likelihood of life difficulties over time.

Eth and Pynoos (1985) state that trauma occurs when an individual is exposed to an overwhelming event resulting in helplessness in the face of intolerable danger, anxiety and instinctual arousal. There is no documen-tation of the general debilitating effects on children's or adolescents' responses to the death of a parent from AIDS. However, it is logical to conclude that the response is stressful and devastating, given the combined effects of the trauma (physical and emotional) and the stigma associated with the disease.

Until recently we have had no systematic way to conceptualize the par-ticular impact parental death has on children. Research on post-traumatic stress syndrome with children offers a partial conceptual framework. The seminal work of Terr (1983, 1985) reveals similarities between the children she studied and the bereaved children and adolescents who we discuss in this chapter. In her pioneer study, Terr interviewed and had follow-up contacts with children who were involved in a bizarre kidnapping incident in Chowchilla, California, in 1983. The children's schoolbus was comman-deered by three men, driven for several hours and then buried with the children still inside. The children eventually dug their way to freedom.

As a result of their involvement in this episode, many of these children evidenced long-term psychological distress, or psychic trauma. Terr (1985) defined psychic trauma as the "emotional condition following from a sudden, unexpected, and intense external blow that overwhelms crucial coping and defense operations, temporarily rendering the individual helpless" (816). She further qualifies this definition by excluding any event, however grievous, that might be reasonably expected in the course of a lifetime, such as sibling births, death of a grandparent or family break-ups. Also, the event must be unanticipated, nonimaginary and piercingly intense—as is the death of a parent from AIDS.

Terr (1985) describes the salient signs and symptoms of post-traumatic stress disorder (PTSD) in children. These include intrusive memories, un-conscious reenactments, startle reactions, recurrent nightmares, fears of re-peated traumas and avoidant or other symptomatic behaviors. Responses to psychic trauma that we found in our observations of both children and adolescent survivors parallel Eth and Pynoos's (1985) findings. They identify deleterious effects on the child's cognition (including memory, school performance and learning), the child's affect, interpersonal relations, impulse control and vegetative function.

COMPREHENSION OF DEATH

Grief-stricken children and adolescents differ in varying respects from their adult counterparts. The capacity of children to sustain sadness or dysphoric affects over time increases with age and ego maturity. Due to a short attention span, children may not be able to participate as fully in bereavement rituals as adults. However, children are subject to the same disturbances of mourning. Complicating our understanding of childhood bereavement is the unsettled question of when they are capable of comprehending death as a finality.

There has been a good deal of speculation regarding the stage of development, reflected in age, of greatest relative risk for unfavorable outcome (e.g. suicide, school failure, inability to cope) following parental death. There is no agreement among studies regarding the ages at which a child is potentially more at risk for long-term adverse consequences of parental bereavement. In general, it appears that early childhood is the period of greatest vulnerability. Schell and Loder-McGough (1977) report that it is not necessary for a child or adolescent to have a realistic concept of death in order to grieve. Further, they suggest that in any case the child or adolescent will react to the separation, and that the main thing to which we all react emotionally in a grief situation is the separation itself.

YOUNGER CHILDREN

In Maria Nagy's (1948) classic work on Hungarian children, she observes three stages in a child's conception of death. In the first stage, from approximately three to five years of age, death is envisioned as a departure, with the dead maintaining an existence somewhere else. The finality of death is denied. In the second stage, between the ages of five and nine, death is personified. Death exists but can be avoided. In the third and final stage, at the age of nine or ten, death is understood to be an inevitable occurrence that happens to all people; it is realistically understood.

Rando (1984) amplifies on this idea by stating that there is more of a cognitive understanding of death and its implications for the child from five to eight. Children of this age are particularly vulnerable, since they understand much about death, but have little coping capacity. Denial is often a prime defense. Children hide their feelings out of concern for appearing babyish. At the same time, they have a great fear of loss of control, exposure and infantile dependence on adults. Often there are also models for children's behavior provided by adults who are unable to express their feelings or grieve openly. The overt behavior may not reflect their inner feelings. These children may be perceived as uncaring, unloving or unaffected, and may not receive the support and comfort they desperately need.

Unless children are given permission and support to deal with their grief, they will shut out feelings. To offset this, children cope by developing a strong fantasy life in an attempt to keep the relationship with the deceased alive. Some children will become self-reliant and helpful in an attempt to inhibit grief, overcompensate for yearning and act out their own needs for care.

PRE-ADOLESCENT CHILDREN

By the age of eight to twelve children have achieved some level of independence. They are, however, still fragile. Parental loss can precipitate the reawakening of feelings of childishness and helplessness and, perhaps, regression to bed-wetting, thumb sucking and so forth. Efforts to control these feelings result in a facade of total independence and coping. Sudden death for a child of this age will usually elicit shock, denial and possibly great anxiety and distress. When death has been anticipated there appears to be less need for extreme denial, although some denial is likely to occur.

Anger may be more easily manifested, since it is a powerful feeling. The child of this age is still unable to accept the finality of her/his personal loss, although the finality and irreversibility of the death in general is recognized. The child may hold on to the relationship in a fantasized, idealized way that can create further problems with the surviving parent, custodial guardian or foster parent. Some children may choose to retreat into some symbolic behavior linked with the deceased parent. They may also try to act grown-up in an attempt to master the pain of their loss and deny their helplessness. In this age group, more than any other, there is a tendency toward fearfulness, phobic behaviors and hypochondriasis.

ADOLESCENTS

Adolescents may feel helpless and frightened and want to retreat to a younger age where there was a sense of being protected. However, they may be compelled by social expectations to act more adult. If the adolescent is expected to comfort family members, conflicts may emerge on two levels, with the adolescent feeling childlike and struggling to cope simultaneously with her/his own grief. For the normally rebellious adolescent the yearning to return to childhood with its symbiosis and powerlessness is often repressed, increasing the risk of pathological mourning.

Anger is more easily expressed than in earlier stages, and can give the adolescent a sense of power to counteract feelings of helplessness. Anger can also fuel depression or be used to inappropriately punish oneself or others for the death. Many adult-like responses to the death on the part of the adolescent will appear, but they will be complicated by typical adolescent problems, including resistance to communicating with adults, overconcern about the acceptability of their responses to others, alienation from adults and peers and lack of knowledge of social expectations. Other developmental issues that compromise the task of mourning for adolescents are problems with separation and dependency, identity, heightened emotionality and sexual conflict (Raphael 1983). In summary, the child's ability to comprehend death as final is essential to grieving. It should be noted that even after a great deal of research there is no unanimity of opinion when this ability emerges.

CLINICAL TREATMENT ISSUES INFLUENCING CHILDHOOD AND ADOLESCENT GRIEF

Although bereavement following the death of a parent from AIDS is very difficult, it need not defeat the individual's efforts at recovery. Clinicians must be aware of the changing series of developmental stages in childhood and adolescent bereavement. The emotional transition and attitudinal change in each stage is the foundation for adaptive role functioning. Denial, designed to maintain the appearance of family well-being despite adverse situational realities, is not uncommon. It may be maladaptive, since new family realities are ignored.

With parental death, a child or adolescent becomes an orphan and may fear that she/he will no longer be provided with food, clothing, shelter and other necessities of life. There is the potential for the child and adolescent to experience significant environmental deprivation following the loss of a parent. In our work, it was reported that some children and adolescents of drug-abusing parents experience significant gain upon the death of the parent. In these cases, grandmothers or other custodial parents provide basic necessities and stability previously unknown or inconsistently available to these youngsters.

Straining the child's ability to cope can be a move to a new residence, loss of income and changes in child-care arrangements before and after the parent's death. Loss of a parent also entails the developmental interference described earlier.

Haan (1977) suggests that a person is either a defender or a coper—that is, an avoider or an approacher. Clinicians report, based on their treatment experiences, that children initially avoid the reality of death, but later actively approach it and achieve integration. Denial and avoidance behavior may contribute to short-term adjustment in the immediate crisis by controlling change-related anxiety (Lazarus 1979). Long-term adjustment, however, demands active approach, recognition and emotional integration of environmental feedback. This agrees with Lazarus's (1979) contention that individuals may display both passive and active modes of coping—both modes contributing to adjustment if they are appropriate to environmental demands.

We interviewed a number of practitioners, in a variety of settings, who are working with bereaved children and adolescents, but we have not studied them in any systematic way. In therapy, children and adolescents report feeling sad, hurt, lonely, angry, frightened, apathetic, confused and numb. These were not the only emotions experienced when a parent died. Based on our interviews and the literature, we will discuss the following grief reactions: guilt, ego constriction, stigma and reunion fantasies. When observed in children and adolescents, these symptoms and behaviors require professional intervention.

GUILT

People generally report feelings of guilt over the death of a loved one, and children and adolescents are no exception. Classical psychoanalytic understanding is that guilt relates to unconscious hostility, in this case directed toward the deceased parent. In this context, the individual feels that her or his own anger was in some way the cause of the parent's death. All children and adolescents harbor angry feelings toward their parents, and at times these may be exhibited in the form of wishes that the parent go away and even die. They may view the parent's death from AIDS as the fulfillment of such wishes and may consider the death to be their own fault. Also, thinking in accordance with the primitive law of talion (an eye for an eye, a tooth for a tooth), the youngster may fear that the dead parent will return to wreak vengeance on the person who caused his death (Gardner 1983).

Gardner (1983) suggests that guilt is used as "an attempt to gain some control over this calamity, for personal control is strongly implied in the idea 'It's my fault.' " (82). In their attempt to understand the events related to AIDS, children of all ages assign responsibility to themselves for events over which they have no control, as in the following examples:

A sixteen-year-old Hispanic adolescent felt guilty because of his mother's death. He told his therapist that he did not treat his mother well, and that if he would have stayed up with her during the night when she was sick, she would not have died. "I felt I did not keep my promise to her."

Another youngster reported:

My mother was in the hospital for a long time. I asked my aunt to visit her, but she always said, "your mother will be home soon." She never got better, and I [an 11-year-old girl] sometimes wish "it was me who died."

Implied in the notion "it's my fault" is the concept of control. The youngsters in the above examples harbor the delusion that they caused their parents' deaths, and presumably they have the ability to bring the parent back to life. The practitioner assisted these children by exploring the beliefs behind their feelings and helped them differentiate between those things in life they could control and those they could not. Learning to assess what realistically could have been known or done for the parent(s) reduces guilt and self-blame. The practitioner supported and encouraged them to form deeper relationships with surviving family members and to develop new friendships. In other families where AIDS occurs, the issue of control may extend to children and adolescents who think they can prevent the deaths of other family members from AIDS.

Therapists can help children and adolescents struggling with guilt by not reinforcing blaming accusations. Sometimes the surviving parent, grandmother, aunt or uncle may produce guilt in the child by comments such as, "What would your mother/father think if she/he were alive to see what you've done?" or "As long as you continue to be bad, your mother or father will not rest peacefully in heaven." Younger children may fear that their parents' ghosts hover over them, waiting for the moment, usually at night, when the ghost can harm or kill the children in retaliation. Suggesting that the spirit of the dead parent is somehow hovering about observing the child or that, although deceased, the parent can still react to what the child does and says, is an attempt to control or get a youngster to comply with caregivers' requests and demands. Even when effective in discipline, this approach can also be the most predictable way of producing pathological guilt (Schowalter et al. 1983).

The guilt induced may not only interfere with the natural mourning process but may also contribute to the formation of various symptoms. For example, one teenager whose father died from AIDS reported going on a stealing spree in the mid-town area of New York. This reflected efforts to reduce his guilt through antisocial behavior; ostensibly he was hoping to get caught and punished. In another example, aggressive acting-out behaviors were reported by two adolescents in their group therapy. They described throwing chairs at a teacher and fellow classmates, and pushing the guards who tried to restrain them as they ran out of the building. The clinician initially helped the adolescents identify their anger and their behaviors in response to these feelings. In subsequent discussion, they were able to link the anger with the guilt they were feeling at the death of their fathers, which, in turn, decreased their acting out at school.

Clinicians can appreciate a variety of ways in which a child or adolescent whose parent has died may become inordinately guilty. Inadequate and/or misguided discussion of the death, or a conspiracy of silence (which is often the case in deaths from AIDS due to the stigma), increase the survivor's vulnerability to self-blame. If parental death is unaddressed in treatment, severe guilt in the child and adolescent survivor may be experienced years after the death. There may also be lifelong risks as a result of the secret and trauma of the parent's death. Eth and Pynoos (1985) found children whose parents committed suicide reacting by developing a major affective disorder when inadequate or misleading discussion took place. Children and adolescents who are grieving after parental death from AIDS are a high-risk group for depression. Feelings of self-blame for the parents' death may contribute to their depressive self-accusations for not having done more.

EGO CONSTRICTION

Since bereavement in children and adolescents may result in a number of emotional, cognitive, behavioral, social and physical problems, the resolution of grief is important. Death for the child and adolescent survivor is a major personal crisis that can have serious consequences for later life. However, it is erroneous to conclude that bereaved survivors will be invariably dysfunctional. Palumbo (1981) admonishes clinicians and theoreticians for making this assumption and suggests part of its origin:

As observers, we tend to structure and select from the observed data those phenomena that have meaning to us or those with which we feel compatible. We make inferences based on our past experiences. We, unwittingly, permit our subjective responses to structure our observations so that they can fit into our preconceptions. In matters as emotion-laden as death, our feelings can interfere powerfully with our scientific stance. Our humanity is engaged by the suffering of another being and we lose our objectivity. (19)

After fully discussing the implications of this stance, Palumbo states unequivocally that "we cannot take for granted that all losses are traumatic and that all trauma necessarily leads to pathological arrest or permanent regression" (31).

Rosenblatt, Walsh and Jackson (1976) describe three related elements that are deemed essential in most cultures for survivors working through a loss, which we apply to an understanding of bereavement in children and adolescents. The three elements are: accepting the loss, altering maladaptive behaviors and expressing feelings associated with the loss.

Accepting the Loss

First, the bereaved person must accept the reality of the loss, that is, she or he must acknowledge that the parent's death has occurred. It is not uncommon for a person to react to the initial news of a death with disbelief, but this reaction must give way to an acknowledgment of the reality of the parent's death before mourning can occur.

As observed in some respondents, custodial parents, such as grandmothers, aunts and foster parents, indicate that cultural norms (for example touching or kissing the deceased) play a significant role in preventing the mourning from taking its natural course. Some families support the view that the expression of feelings is somehow primitive or improper, and that those who respond to pain with composure are more admirable. Such observations as seeing a grandmother or surviving parent cut off their feelings or not crying, and hearing compliments about this behavior, can have a powerful influence on the youngster and inhibit the mourning process. Some boys in Latino families have been encouraged to "be brave" and told that "crying is not for grown-up men like you." The clinician's task is to allow the grieving child to express her/his painful feelings in a supportive context and to express the feelings of hurt rather than to minimize or deny them.

Altering Maladaptive Behaviors

Second, behaviors associated with the deceased parent must be altered. Extinction of behaviors that are no longer adaptive is essential to the process of working through grief. If a surviving parent, custodial grandmother or aunt, for instance, continues to maintain the room of a deceased parent as if the deceased person were alive, she is failing to adapt to the changed reality. Inner-city families may not be able to create such a monument, due to housing constrictions, but children in these families have revealed other ways in which the deceased is memorialized. A seventeen-year-old girl discussed with her therapist a birthday party the family had for her deceased mother, three months after the mother's death. The family coaxed the girl into participating, and she joined in feeling that she would betray her mother if she did not attend. Furthermore, she did not want to cause discomfort for her extended family.

Expressing Feelings Associated with the Loss

Third, feelings of guilt and anger, and other emotions associated with the loss, must dissipate. Post-death rituals and the viewing of the body provide an appropriate setting and occasion for the direct expression of the strong emotions being felt. Yet often children are not permitted to attend funerals or other ceremonies. This is not to say that all emotions can or will be expressed at the funeral, but it does provide the beginning for the mourning process. For most bereaved people, time and the grieving process serve to lessen the intensity of emotion surrounding a death. When this does not occur, an individual continues to react to thoughts of the deceased with intense and painful emotions.

The tendency to view children as somehow immune from bereavement can cause a profound ego constriction. The child and adolescent may shun intense emotion; suffer the loss of the omnipotence of youth, causing the narrowing of life choices; and develop cognitive difficulties (Eth & Pynoos

1985). We have found that many bereaved children whose parent(s) died from AIDS have difficulties in school. Some children have mild symptoms of learning disabilities, reading problems and forgetting assignments and schedules. These may be due to the intrusion of memories and reminders of the parent's death, which interfere with concentration. Some adolescents have coped with their loss in school through drinking binges, truancy, hitting younger children and inanimate objects and intimidating teachers.

Teachers are valuable links in the total bereavement recovery. Frequently, they are unaware of the death, and do not understand the negative and sometimes violent behavior children and adolescents exhibit as a way of coping with parental loss. Bereaved children and adolescents characteristically engage in conscious and unconscious attempts to manage the stress. Practitioners can provide consultation to teachers and support to the bereaved child during the early transition period. These interventions can provide an anchor as the child's or adolescent's life is disrupted by changes in their living situation and financial resources and by custodial conflicts.

School is particularly significant for the bereaved adolescent who is dealing with autonomy, body image, sex roles and peer relationships during a time of grievous loss. It is important to allow adolescents to maximize their own sense of control. Participation in a group work treatment program at school is an effective way to achieve this goal.

Children in our study sustained a parent's death and often suffered concomitant losses of siblings, aunts, uncles and others from AIDS. In spite of children's and adolescents' tendency to react less strongly to death than adults, parental death is likely to result in depression. In severe cases of depression youngsters can become apathetic. They lose interest in the world and appear to be insensitive to stimuli, both internal and external.

The case of Charlie clearly illustrates these dynamics:

Charlie, a ten-year-old African-American child, had been brought to the Family Service Center by his aunt who complained about his withdrawal, his crying when he thought no one was paying attention to him as well as his manifesting clinging behavior. She described him as a different person since his mother's death two months ago. As the worker accompanied Charlie to the office, he was impressed with how sad the youngster seemed.

Mr. Jones, the social worker, encouraged Charlie to tell him how things were going, but the youngster responded with stoic silence. The worker respected this silence, but periodically made comments informing Charlie that he thought he seemed very sad, and that the worker knew his teachers were complaining about his behavior at school, and that his aunt was very concerned about him. It was not until the worker commented that he thought this was connected to Charlie's mother's death, that he noticed the first overt reaction. Two tears ran down Charlie's cheek, as he turn to face the worker for the first time.

Charlie slowly told the worker that he was now living with his aunt. In the past, going to his aunt's house was great fun. Living with his mother in the nearby housing project allowed him to play with his friends, but his aunt always made it a special occasion when he went there. He talked about his last birthday, his tenth, when his mother took seven of his friends to his aunt's and they had a great time playing and eating, and he got a lot of presents.

Based on the information the worker received from Charlie's aunt, he commented that it was close to his tenth birthday that his mother became ill. Charlie agreed, saying that she had lost a lot of weight, but immediately after his birthday party she went to the hospital for the first time. He had to live with his aunt while his mother was hospitalized. He wasn't happy because he worried about his mother. He was in school when his mother went to the hospital the second time. The school social worker called him out of class and told him that his aunt called and would pick him up after school. When she did he could tell that something was wrong. He knows that she had been crying, which was something that she never did. She hugged him close and slowly told him that his mother was very sick. He told the worker that it all started when she had a trans—. The worker asked if he meant "transfusion." Charlie said yes, that's what it was, and she got some bad blood then. He went on to say that his aunt mentioned that no one could say whether his mother would live, but she assured him that his mother wanted him to live with her, and that she would take care of him because she loved him dearly.

With help from the worker, Charlie talked about his mother's death and how cold her body was in the open casket. He remembers that lots of people came to the funeral, and he also talked about how difficult it was to move his things to his aunt's house shortly after. The worker empathized with Charlie and told him that it was hard to have a parent whom he loves die. He said that children always feel sad and frequently ask many questions about what will happen to them. He then asked Charlie what worried him the most.

With tears running down his cheeks, Charlie said that he was worried about two things. At night he wakes up seeing his mother who is very skinny and hardly able to talk. He hears her whispering to him "I love you," and he gets very scared. His second worry is that his aunt might die also and that he would be all alone. He knows that she isn't sick, but she is all he has now and doesn't know who would care for him or what he would do. The worker commented that other kids have similar worries. Charlie recalled that the mother of two of his friends at school died from AIDS. They went to live with their aunt, but she died last week. Tom and Jimmy had to leave school and moved to Brooklyn to live with another aunt.

The worker reached over to touch Charlie's hands and confirm how difficult it is to be alone. He told Charlie that many children have these same worries when there is a death in the family, and suggested that he and Charlie could talk together over the next few months and think about this and other worries. Charlie agreed that it would be helpful, because although he loves his aunt and she talks to him all the time, he hasn't been able to tell her what really worries him.

In extreme cases, clinicians need to be vigilant, since bereaved adolescents may engage in self-destructive behavior and/or attempt suicide. A practitioner described to us an adolescent who resisted engaging in safer sex. The clinician explored the beliefs behind this behavior and learned that the adolescent felt that if she got AIDS, she could rejoin her mother. Furman (1974) states that elements of identification may be present in such cases, as well as attempts to reunite with the dead parent.

STIGMA

Although they are experiencing intense, painful feelings surrounding the death, the overwhelming majority of the children and adolescents in treatment have not shared their reactions with anyone prior to being referred to the clinician.

Very few survivors of a death from AIDS emerge without some sense of stigma. In our review, we found three different interrelated aspects of stigma that play a role in the mourning of children and adolescents. They are: (1) the involuntary acceptance of negative attitudes about oneself (stigmatization); (2) the disrepute associated with death (general stigma); and (3) the specific dishonor attributed to persons with AIDS and their survivors (stigma of association with AIDS).

Stigmatization

Stigmatization is a belief in and an internalization of negative attitudes toward the self. This negative focus results in a redefinition of the self as worthy of hatred and rejection, not only by the reference group but by the self as well. Goffman (1963) has referred to this process as the spoiling of identity. In the case of bereaved children and adolescents, this new, damaged and devalued self is further handicapped by perceptions of difference from the rest of society, of failure to meet its standards and of inferiority.

The consequences of stigmatization are usually unconscious. The spoiling of one's identity and the internalization of stigma change the way in which the bereaved person approaches and deals with others.

General Stigma

The concept of stigma recognized by Parkes (1980) is the attitude of society toward the newly bereaved person. As people avoid the youngster or become uncomfortable in his or her presence, it is as if in some way the bereaved child or adolescent becomes tainted by death.

Children and adolescents who survive any death feel uncertainty and shame. They frequently dread returning to school after the funeral or other rituals, wishing to avoid the questions posed or likely to be posed by their peers. Questions about death from AIDS may be extremely frightening, because of the stigma complicated by the extant uncertainties and contradictions. Conversely, children may be avoided or subjected to anger or humor bordering on ridicule from their peers.

Stigma Directed at PWAs and their Survivors

The stigma attached to death from AIDS magnifies the emotional trauma experienced by bereaved children and adolescents. AIDS is equated with being immoral and untouchable (see Chapters 2 and 3).

Compounding both children's and adolescents' dilemma, this stigmatized death damages the network of family, friends and social supports. Although all bereaved people are somewhat socially stigmatized and may experience altered social relationships, deaths from AIDS, like deaths by murder and suicide, are more stigmatizing and traumatic than others. Lacking supports and experiencing callous responses to a parent's death are not desirable for coping with the grief process. It is common for these bereaved children to experience—often based on the reality of the way they are treated by others—feelings of abandonment, helplessness and frustration in reaction to their parent's death from AIDS, far beyond the level normally experienced by bereaved children.

Feelings of estrangement, primarily from adolescent peer groups, are most pronounced. Social isolation is exacerbated by prejudice and fear of contagion. Isolation is further compounded by misunderstanding of socially unacceptable or acting-out behaviors and prolonged absences from school. Many adolescents are alienated from their peers as they assume the roles of caregiver and surrogate parent for younger siblings during a parent's illness and death. Isolation, when prolonged, will intensify the child's dependence on adults in the environment or result in deviant behavior to gain attention. In an adolescent, isolation may encroach on age-specific developmental tasks, such as the renegotiation of separation and individuation. Not knowing how to deal with the demands of the caregiving role, the adolescent survivor may say little about it. Silence may reflect fear of angering people in the environment and of provoking further reprisal.

Alienation and isolation, resulting from stigma, influence the course of grieving. When they become protracted, the behavioral responses may lead to lifelong difficulties in interpersonal behavior. The double-edged sword of a parent's death and the stigma associated with AIDS results in the widespread experience of a conspiracy of silence. The difficulty in returning to a normal life following parental death, and the fear of other tragedies, such as the death of a second parent or another family member, are issues that confront inner-city, disenfranchised children. Loneliness and sadness after a parent's death from AIDS are often the emotional aftermath of a frightening and overwhelming experience.

Practitioners have stated that they observed some adolescent survivors "growing up overnight" after their parents' deaths. Often adolescents "parent" their younger siblings, and frequently forego their own grief. Sometimes teenagers go to extreme lengths in overprotecting their younger sisters and brothers to shield them from the insensitive remarks made by peers. A seventeen-year-old girl related how she kept her younger brothers home from school saying they were sick. This was her way of protecting them from being singled out by other children in their class who referred to them as "AIDS kids." Many times a favored position in the family is the role of "rescuer." Playing this role allays underlying feelings of helplessness and anxiety.

The following case illustrates many of the above clinical issues.

Jerry's grandmother, Mrs. B., brought him to the cardiac clinic when she came for her monthly checkup. She casually mentioned being concerned about him to the nurse. When the nurse expressed interest, Mrs. B. revealed additional details, which prompted a referral to the social worker.

Mrs. B. revealed that for the past two years Jerry had difficulty sleeping. He frequently woke up crying, and complaining about frightening nightmares. Recently, he has been having more conflicts with his younger sister, at whom he lashed out at the slightest provocation. His teachers contacted Mrs. B. and complained about his poor peer relationships and his lack of interest in school activities.

On further exploration, the worker learned that Jerry's father, a former IV drug user, and his mother died within six months of each other, about a year after a diagnosis of AIDS. Mrs. B. was the closest relative and became the custodial parent. She talked with strong emotions about the difficulties of this role. She began to cry as she recalled watching her daughter and son-in-law deteriorate physically and mentally. At the time she had little information about AIDS or other tangible resources to support her caregiving role.

When they died, Mrs. B. said, she consciously decided that she would forget the painful experience. "At the time I made up mind to dedicate myself to caring for Jerry and his sister and to make their lives comfortable."

In response to the worker's gentle probing, Mrs. B. indicated that Jerry was eight years old at the time of their deaths and seemed to have been unaffected by the illness and death of his parents. At times when they were feeling strong, his parents spent lots of time with him. They took him to places where he might have fun, and they made every effort to give him tangible evidence of their love and affection. Both parents and Mrs. B. thought he could not understand the illness or the meaning of death. Consequently, they told him nothing and he did not ask any questions. Both the wake and funerals were very simple and Jerry did not attend. Mrs. B. had arranged for a friend to care for him and his sister on those days.

Mrs. B. felt that both grandchildren had made good adjustments to their parents' deaths. She had not been concerned until she began hearing about Jerry's behavior at school. It was the principal who suggested that he might be having a problem. The worker attempted several times to make the link between his parents' illnesses and deaths and Jerry's behaviors, but Mrs. B. did not respond. She agreed for the worker to see Jerry alone, and they all met for a brief time before Jerry's interview with the worker.

As soon as the worker asked how things were going, Jerry said that he missed his parents. He talked about all the good times they had as he fought back the tears. The worker spoke gently and soothingly to him, convincing him that it was all right if he felt like crying. When the question was posed as to when he missed his parents the most, Jerry told that he felt cheated last Christmas when he received only one present. "When my mother and father were alive, we always had lots of food and candy, a big tree covered with balls and lots of presents underneath. Grandma keeps saying that we have to have a quiet Christmas. I wish my parents were still alive, but I can't tell that to my grandmother." Further exploration revealed that Jerry did indeed know more details about his parents' death than his grandmother suspected, but he also had many questions. It was clear that he wanted to talk about them and simply to think aloud about the good times he had with his parents. Jerry also communicated that, although nothing had been said, his grandmother would disapprove if he talked about them, and would be hurt and angry. "This is why I talk to my parents sometimes when I go to bed. It helps, but sometimes I get scared that they may want to take me to be with them." The worker invited Jerry to return and Mrs B. agreed to bring him in on a weekly basis. She also stated she was ready to talk to someone at the clinic about her role as a grandparent.

In the subsequent fifteen interviews, Jerry repeatedly asked many questions about the disease and revealed how his parents looked so skinny. He wondered if they had gained weight since they died. He talked about missing his parents and brought in pictures the family took at the zoo about six months before his mother died. Jerry revealed many early memories and also talked about secrets his mother told him and his sister. He felt his grandmother was talking more about his parents. With great pride, he revealed how the teachers at school praised him for getting good marks. "I feel better even though I know my Mom and Dad are not coming back. I know they can see me from heaven and know what's happening to me."

The effects of Jerry's parents' death on his family (grandmother and sister), as well as his reactions, are similar to those reported by a number of clinicians working with bereaved children. Symptoms of stress and trauma are likely to occur when parents die. Attempts at denial and suppression of sad and frightening feelings are not uncommon. Helping the child, as well as the caregiver, to acknowledge and communicate their feelings is a beginning toward coping with a major loss such as the death of a parent.

Failure to mourn is usually related to the family's conscious efforts, as in Jerry's case, to avoid any sharing of memories and emotions related to the deceased. It was striking to observe how both Jerry and his grandmother quickly released a lot of pent-up feelings in regard to the deaths. As is true in the case of any treatment procedure, timing is important. When helping the bereaved to bring out grief reactions, the clinician must be sensitive to the defenses holding back the discharge of feelings. In the case of Jerry, he was comfortable in expressing his feelings; when he felt powerless, his only way to discharge his emotions was through provocation or through nightmares.

Despite Mrs B.'s earlier coping through denial she became an important ally in the brief clinical work with Jerry. She also gained much satisfaction from his change to a more content and better adjusted preadolescent.

REUNION FANTASIES

In order to cope with and master their world, children create defensive fantasies of reunion and restitution. These fantasies are common in bereavement at all ages. They are an attempt to suppress or limit the magical power of hidden wishes. Much as the witch-doctor does with his rites and spells, children use words or ritualistic games to protect themselves from harm and death. For bereaved children this activity also serves to recapture the lost parent.

For children five years of age and less, grief responses are quite variable (Raphael 1983). Many do not understand the death fully and ask seemingly inappropriate questions immediately afterwards. Practitioners working with younger children concur with Rando (1984) that children often show a degree of bewilderment and exhibit some regressive behavior by becoming clinging and demanding. They are likely to inquire repeatedly about the whereabouts of the deceased parent(s) and demand to know why they have not returned and what they are doing. There is obvious yearning for the parent's return and angry protest when it does not occur. There is often anger with the deceased parent(s) for desertion and for the resulting chaos in family life.

Some children suffer multiple bereavements of both parents and significant others across generations in their family of origin. As a result, they lose the security of the relationships and a familiar environment. Their sense of security may be totally disrupted, giving rise to concerns for their own survival. Preoccupation with the deceased feelings of longing and sadness are common. To cope, these children may develop a strong fantasy life in an attempt to keep the relationship with the deceased alive.

Many times well-meaning adults avoid communicating to children and adolescents their real views regarding the parent's death. They may tell them about a blissful afterlife in heaven without any conviction that this is so. While the intention is to offer comfort and solace, this produces both unnecessary confusion and a wish to rejoin the parent(s), since children are in need of a secure and trusting relationship. The child's reactions can be balanced by openness among the extended family about the death and by the provision of a genuinely supportive relationship.

In the case of a sixteen-year-old Hispanic adolescent, depression, combined with a reunion fantasy, produced a powerful urge, to commit suicide in the hope of being buried next to her mother and rejoining her in heaven. This case is distinctive because of the relative ease with which this adolescent girl readily engaged in the therapeutic process. The mourning was accomplished mainly through the process of interpretation of her behavior and reassuring her that she would be taken care of by her extended family. Some children and adolescents view their parent's death as an abandonment and fear that the remaining parent or guardian will either die or abandon them as well.

The focus of this adolescent's therapy, as discussed in the following example, dwelled on the mourning process during the entire eleven months of treatment.

Rose was in group treatment with the social worker for about two months before she was referred to a mental health clinic in the neighborhood. The group's focus was to identify, explore and discuss issues of interest to teenagers. During a group session, Rose seemed preoccupied and uninterested in participation. After the session, the social worker learned that Rose's mother had died a week before from AIDS. Not being able to offer ongoing individual sessions, the worker told Rose about the neighborhood satellite clinic. The program offered both individual and family treatment. A referral was initiated and Rose's aunt was amenable to accompanying Rose for her first visit.

Rose began the interview by telling the worker that her mother had died of AIDS. She recalled that since she was 10 years old she knew her mother was a prostitute. Rose shared several stories that her mother related to her before she left the house in the early evening. Rose remembered her mother preparing dinner, spending time talking and watching a favorite TV show before she left in the evening. Her aunt would tuck her into bed on those evenings. Rose recalled her mother being home in the morning and helping her to get ready for school. The "family secret" was well respected by the extended family members who shared in Rose's upbringing. Rose said that she felt no shame, since several relatives of her schoolmates were also prostitutes and there seemed to be no particular resentment directed at her.

"When my mother became ill two years ago I was not immediately sure what was wrong. As my mother's condition worsened, I learned from an aunt that my mother had developed AIDS. From my health class at school I knew that this was a serious illness and that my mother would probably not survive. I began spending as much time as I could with my mother, caring for some of her physical needs but primarily talking about our lives together and about my mother's childhood on a farm in the Midwest. Many of the stories were romanticized, full of pictures of freedom, wide open spaces, riding horses and having a strong sense of community. My mother talked of her disappointment about not being able to realize her long-held dream of taking me to her home, so I could experience the idyllic childhood that she cherished." Rose did not recall it being said specifically, but she had the sense that life after death would be exactly like the descriptions her mother recalled of her childhood, that is "being free." A tone of sadness followed these memories.

The worker conveyed how sad it is when a mother dies and how helpful it can be to share one's feelings of sadness with another person. Rose expressed her fears of being alone and recalled the night her mother died. "We both had a good time talking together and reminiscing about funny experiences we shared. I was very sad and cried a great deal at the wake and funeral. There was a good feeling, however, knowing that my mother was in heaven and that ultimately I would join her there. As time passed, I began to miss my mother more and more and began thinking that reuniting with my mother would be the perfect solution to my loneliness." Rose was adamant that she wasn't thinking about suicide when she took the pills but saw it as a way of going to be with her mother. "My aunt discovered my plan and began spending more time with me, shopping and talking together. I love her very much, but she is not my mother."

The worker encouraged Rose to talk about her feeling sad and lonely, and to express her fears about the changes in her life since her mother had died. A theme that reasserted itself again and again in ongoing weekly sessions was Rose's feelings of loneliness and her recollection of the happy times she had had with her mother. Rose related a dream she had about her mother: "I woke up, crying and feeling all alone." The worker supported her feelings, saying, "It's hard not to miss someone whom you love and felt close to."

Rose later asked whether she would still be brave if she cried. The worker said certainly, "One has nothing to do with the other." The worker asked if sometimes she held back her tears when she felt like crying. She said, "Yes, all the time, except when I talk to my mother about going to live with her in heaven." She paused, looked at the worker intently, and said, "I can also cry in here."

Within less than a year, Rose said that she was less afraid and that she now found comfort when she was able to talk about her mother. She talks about her mother with her family and friends and feels less alone. When she talks to the worker she holds on to a locket, which her mother gave her and feels good. She now takes pleasure from her school performance and her outside activities. In one of her sessions, Rose said, "I have never talked to anyone like this before. I know that there is something missing in my life, but you have helped me to think that there is so much I have to remember which makes me feel OK and warm inside."

Rose is a classic example of many adolescents and children who believe that their parents are in heaven and, when feeling lonely, want to go there and rejoin their parents. For some, the reunion fantasy not only serves to recapture the deceased parent(s) but also reverses the death. The reunion also reduces the feelings of loneliness and pain experienced upon the death of a parent. Feelings of hopelessness over the irreversibility of the event, and a sense of personal guilt for having failed to do more, as in the case of Rose, can precipitate negative consequences.

Clinicians need to evaluate the overall resilience of adolescents, since depressive feelings or sadness connected with bereavement can quickly escalate into a clinical depression. Thoughts of one's own death are rarely far from consciousness in the minds of many of the bereaved. Besides wishing to rejoin her mother, Rose posed other questions to the worker as Rose wondered about the nature of death. Will the afterlife be anything like contemporary existence? Will death solve my problems and erase all my concerns? Attention to these preoccupations is imperative, as unanswered questions may inspire suicidal ideation or behaviors.

In order for adolescents to work through the death of a parent, their childhood, including infantile ties, must be relinquished. A part of this process involves the vivid and passionate reliving of early experiences and attachments. One can assume that the return in memory and feelings to the past carries both special urgency and pain for an adolescent who has lived through the death of a parent.

FORESHORTENED SENSE OF THE FUTURE

Terr (1985) describes children who survive traumatic events as developing a "philosophical pessimism" about their own future. They believe that they will die young or express doubt that they will live past certain "landmark" birthdays, such as the sixteenth, eighteenth, or twenty-first. Others have suggested that the ability to orient oneself to long-range, future goals or interests, and thus one's ability to tolerate frustration depends on having had successes in the past (Silber & Wortman 1984; Tooley 1978).

The children of the Chowchilla kidnapping were reported by Terr to be severely pessimistic. We were informed about similar attitudes by clinicians working with children and adolescents bereaved by AIDS. Some of these children live in high-crime, inner-city communities. Their pessimistic views of life and forshortened sense of the future, inspired previously by dangerous environmental conditions, the absence of successful role models and limited experiences with personal success, are compounded with the death from AIDS. The fact that a cure for this disease is yet to be developed contributes further to their pessimism.

ADVOCATING FOR CHILDREN'S PERMANENCE

AIDS has caused the deaths of parents, brothers, sisters and extended family members of children and adolescents who do not themselves have AIDS. Notable efforts have been made to respond to the needs of children orphaned by the deaths of parents from AIDS and extended family members. Foster care and extended family care programs have been initiated; competent and dedicated people who care about children's well-being have offered their services. Secure and permanent homes are desperately needed for these non-infected children, many of whom are African-American or Hispanic. The need to maintain, expand and replicate quality efforts has been recognized, but there is room for many more creative ideas and programs.

Many children who have experienced early separations and neglect may be distrustful of adults and may display angry, rejecting postures. They appear to demand more understanding, especially as they confront their grief. Both children and adolescents may confront grief reactions and behaviors associated with crack and intravenous drug use on the part of mothers and fathers. They may not be the "cute" and "adorable" children potential foster parents request. The recruitment of foster homes for AIDS survivors will require intensive and consistent efforts. This community of bereaved and orphaned children demands immense patience and trust that may stretch the limits of potential foster parents.

Specialized in-service training is needed to prepare foster parents for the challenges posed by this cohort of children and adolescents. Ideally, education—buttressed by ongoing support and consultation—can prepare foster parents for unexpected crises, help them understand behaviors related to grief and mourning, reduce the anxiety, fear and prejudice that surround AIDS and help correct misconceptions and stereotypes (Anderson 1990). It is hoped that this will produce more permanency in foster care and not create a series of different placements due to lack of understanding of behaviors that can be recognized and given realistic attention. It is important for practitioners to be able to set realistic goals for helping families cope with bereaved children and reduce further disruption in their lives.

GROUP AND INDIVIDUAL TREATMENT

Post-grieving assistance to children and adolescents is most appropriately given by their surviving parent or surrogate caregiver. Our observations lead us to conclude that parents and surrogate caregivers are themselves grieving as a consequence of the death and non-supportive elements in the environment. The task for professionals is to provide an emotional climate that will enable children and adolescents to avail themselves of group and/or individual treatment to facilitate the expression and resolution of grief.

Help for bereaved children that is described in the professional literature has focused on individual treatment (Greenberg 1975; Savin 1987). The literature on treatment of bereaved children whose parents have died from AIDS is nonexistent. In individual treatment, as in group process, mourning proceeds with the awareness, comprehension and acknowledgment of death. A gradual decathexis occurs as a withdrawal of investment in the person takes place, as well as a wish to live for life's pleasure. Through the process of identification, the child's ties with the loved object become internalized even as there is recognition that there will be no further good memories to be garnered.

Support groups are reported to be helpful for children who have suffered loss through parental divorce (Bonkowski, Bequette & Boomhower 1984; Epstein & Bordin 1985). Adapting these models, Masterman and Reams (1988) developed support groups for bereaved preschool and school-age children whose parents had died from non-AIDS deaths. Given the shock to the family system, and especially to the surviving parent or custodial/surrogate parent, Masterman and Reams (1988) found a supportive type of intervention helpful to facilitate normal grieving and to prevent pathological grief reactions.

Practitioners whom we interviewed felt successful in utilizing the group model with adolescents, but less so with younger and latency-age bereaved children. Lack of funds to provide transportation and time needed by the significant other to accompany the child to the community-based mental health center or the hospital contributed to the lack of success. In family service agencies, practitioners reported the successful use of a combination of direct work, extensive play therapy and activity groups with preadolescent children, who have a greater tendency to process issues through symbolic play than verbally.

Clinicians working in school settings relate limited success in utilizing time-limited groups with latency-age children who are released from their regular classes with no negative consequences. These clinicians use Gordon's (1978) model, which emphasizes stories with themes centered around death and mourning. The objective is to have the children identify with the main character and to have them consider the therapeutic resolution achieved by the main character as a strategy they might utilize. Questions are asked by the group leader to reemphasize the main points and help the children draw parallels between the protagonist and themselves or their own lives. Themes include: how the parent died, fear of the self or the remaining parent or surrogate parent dying, anger at the parent who died, separation anxiety, what it is like where the deceased parent is now, getting along with siblings, memories and dreams, fear and sadness and termination of the group.

Although the data are limited, parents and custodial caregivers report a decrease in behavior problems at home and school and increased communication with their children around bereavement issues not previously discussed. This is not the case with the adolescent group members. Their behavior problems may be attributable to normative issues of separation and independent striving.

IMPLICATIONS FOR PRACTICE

The challenges facing professionals working with bereaved children and adolescents are enormous. The death of a parent or significant other is one of the most emotionally stressful events that can happen to a child or adolescent. The resolution of grief is important to avoid a number of emotional, behavioral, cognitive, social and physical problems that can emerge and invariably lead to dysfunction. Integration and assimilation of the death is a slow process for children and adolescents. They can complete the grief work, achieve integration and develop added dimensions to their personality with structured guidance and emotional support from adults.

Practitioners working with bereaved children and adolescents should consider the following:

• Grieving children and adolescents are not unlike adults who grieve.
• Developmental capacities and age-related concerns need consideration.
• Initial denial is adaptive in the early crisis state and only maladaptive if it persists.

Children and adolescents will engage in behaviors that reflect their search for the lost parent or loved one. Since they will not succeed in this endeavor, a period of withdrawal is inevitable before they can proceed to develop and appreciate a substitute attachment (Dersheimer 1990). Surrogate parents will need to be educated and supported while the bereaved children and adolescents go through this withdrawal. The behavior of surrogate parents who react to the withdrawal with overt disappointment, anger or a corresponding withdrawal precludes successful integration by the youngsters.

At the same time, children and adolescents must form and retain an inner image of the person who has died. Practitioners can help them develop images that are realistic, devoid of superhuman or magical qualities and that will permit them to develop appropriate attachments and maintain a good self-image.

Adolescents whose physical, intellectual and future development epitomizes living and growth will be particularly vulnerable to conflicts stemming from arrested grieving. Death is by nature unreal. Their acceptance of the death of a loved one, with all its implications, may take a longer, more convoluted route. Educational approaches that prepare them and their significant others for the uneven course of the grieving process will be extremely useful. Willingness to stay with them during the pain and sadness and to assist with the complexities of their development will in itself be supportive, while providing the requisite climate for confronting and coping with their pain and suffering.

It is our belief that immediate and timely intervention with children and adolescents mourning the deaths of parents from AIDS can mitigate some of the negative, lifelong responses to this overwhelming trauma. The importance of interagency liaison and aggressive outreach, so as to engage and ensure continuing treatment compliance, is essential to engage families in mental health treatment.

In planning intervention and appraising its success, one must take into account changing intrapersonal, interpersonal and situational demands. Intrapersonal factors, such as failure to work through a parent's death in adolescence or in later life, might cause attitudinal difficulties with regard to marriage and the willingness to make personal commitment. Changing interpersonal circumstances after a death in the family, such as living with a surviving parent (many times HIV-infected) or substitute parental figure, might negatively affect limit-setting and adjustment (Hetherington, Stanley-Hagan and Anderson 1989). Situational factors, such as multiple deaths, preclude full adjustment, and may require intensive or long-term care before integration and recovery can be considered successful. Based on our clinical observations, early explorations of these events is important for recovery.

By maintaining as much stability and consistency as possible, surrogate parents and clinicians can enhance a sense of control and mastery over the inner and outer upheaval that children and adolescents experience. Encouraging the expression of painful and ambivalent feelings associated with the death of parents can help correct distorted fantasies and facilitate an ability to mourn.

CHAPTER 5

Intervening with Women

AIDS constitutes a legacy of loss. Death from AIDS presents a unique set of problems with physical, psychological, sociological, moral and even political implications for women, an emerging group of silent grievers. Persons with AIDS, having been alienated for an extended period of time, often return home to their loved ones to live out the remaining days of their lives. Each person in the family system is touched by the illness and death of its member. Women, however, assume greater long-term responsibility than men for care of family members with AIDS. Women with a family member ill with AIDS not only represent the "worried well," they are often not well themselves. They are predominantly poor people, members of families in conflict, disruption and disintegration, alienated and socially stigmatized.

Theorists and researchers have examined the experience of AIDS within the family system (Macklin 1989; Walker 1987). Most clinicians agree that the family system is the primary healer for persons who are grieving, and that members turn to each other for comfort, understanding and grief resolution. We believe that sexism and racism have resulted in the neglect of women as they shoulder the role of survivors. When their sons, daughters, husbands, lovers or grandchildren are infected and die of the disease, they continue to minister to the family. This is the case either when the loved one has been an ongoing member of the family or when the loved one has reentered the family system after being diagnosed with AIDS.

This chapter addresses clinical practice intervention with bereaved women whose family members have died from AIDS. While women's cultural training or socialization is diverse from country to country, race to race and from ethnic group to ethnic group, women are all socialized to continue to work, care for their children and maintain their homes as they seek to transcend their attachment and loss. We examine the pivotal roles women as survivors experience as they grieve their loved ones' death from AIDS. The meaning of attachment and affiliation to a woman's identity may well grow out of her involvement with others. Her sense of self may be organized primarily around her ability to make and then to maintain affiliations and relationships (Miller & Ingram 1976).

Drawing from the literature on trauma and survivorship, we generalize the findings to the experience of women balancing their grief on a continuum from despair and hopelessness to integration. Chronic sorrow enables some women to challenge the adverse effects of death from AIDS. Case studies illustrate the range and differences of women as they face the deaths of loved ones from AIDS.

OVERVIEW

Traumatic experiences often have immediate psychiatric consequences. Sometimes, however, the manifestations of the trauma are, or seem to be, delayed. Delayed onset can be said to occur when an individual at first appears to respond adaptively to traumatic stress but then develops a wide range of stressful reactions after an asymptomatic latency period. The trigger for the sudden surfacing of the stress may be an event that echoes some symbolic or stressful life event, such as a death from AIDS.

When a woman experiences the irrevocable loss of her husband, lover, baby, adult child or grandchild, her basic sense of self is shattered. She has not only lost a relationship but also a sense of who she is. Unless, or until, she attains a new sense of herself and develops a new identity, she remains frozen in her outdated self, grieving, mourning and depressed (Silverman 1981). If she is to emerge from these shadows, a woman must find ways to deal with her loss. Although this loss reflects a permanent impact on her sense of self, there is the potential for change, adaptation and the development of new relationships and another identity.

It is impossible to overemphasize the profound emotional, physical and psychological impact AIDS has on women survivors of all ages, races and cultures as they mourn the deaths of their loved ones.

- The mother learns of her own HIV infection after her child is born with AIDS. Her guilt over transmitting AIDS to her baby and her worries over the care of her two young children are profound.

- The grandmother is working on custody of her grandchildren as she is concurrently parenting and mourning the death of her second daughter to AIDS.

- A middle-aged mother weeps as she tells other mothers in her weekly support group how she vividly recalls her son's frail, limp body during the last few weeks prior to his death, while expressing relief that she was able to meet his last request of dying at home.

- A mother tells her three teenage children that their father died of AIDS and that she fears her own potential for being HIV-infected.

- The mother tells her son that his seventy-five-year-old father died of AIDS from a blood transfusion, and speaks of her uncontrollable anger at the medical profession for not taking necessary precautions.

- The mother whose eight year old daughter, a hemophiliac, died two years ago cannot "go on" spending hours alone in her daughter's room and avoiding her other two children and husband.

To assist in the healing of pain for women who have spent many years nurturing and caring for children, or as a caregiver for dying spouses, lovers, young or adult children, is a challenging task for mental health practitioners. The goal of clinical practice, in each situation, is to help women cope with and resolve the accumulated stresses and the emotional havoc and pain that death evokes. The practitioner must understand the dynamics of "off-time" loss and chronic sorrow that women experience and how women grieve.

OFF-TIME LOSS

To understand better the reaction of women who are attempting to resolve the intense distress caused by their loved ones' deaths from AIDS, the therapist must understand where these women are in the developmental life cycle, and that major nonnormative losses tend to have a profound impact, upsetting the normal rhythm of life. How the woman has reacted to illness and loss (Carter & McGoldrick 1988; Moss 1984; Herz 1980) is an important issue to elicit in treatment. Exploration can promote discussion of the woman's experience prior to the diagnosis and death from AIDS, including relevant splits, alliances, collusions and cutoffs (McGoldrick & Gerson 1985).

In the treatment of loss and grief, we are dealing with an unwritten natural law: the more attached an individual is to someone, the deeper the grief will be when that person dies. For a young child, life has only just begun, and when it is interrupted by death from AIDS, survivors experience a tragedy.

Given the traditional role expectations for women in our culture, an older mother of the person who has died from AIDS is at a time in her life when she has just relinquished caretaking responsibilities. As a result she may experience several emotional reactions: a sense of relief, loss, freedom or success at having been a good parent. Prior to the death, she must readapt and resume a former role. Finally, after the death, a resurgence of unfulfilled dreams, hopes, and expectations for the future can emerge.

The most distressing and long-lasting of all griefs, as noted earlier, is the death of a child. In many ways the death of a child represents or symbolizes the death of the self. Garfield (1979) states: "It is to the parents of a dead child that fate delivers the severest blow. We fear for our children as we fear for ourselves. Never have we lived or loved enough. Death always comes too soon" (316).

Sanders (1980), in comparing reactions to the loss of a spouse, child and parent, found that those who experienced the death of a child revealed more intense grief reactions of somatic types, greater depression as well as anger, and greater guilt with accompanying feelings of despair than did those bereaved who had experienced the death of either a spouse or parent.

According to a number of developmental theorists, death is a salient issue for mid-life adults. Failing health, deaths of parents, loss of close friends and changes in physical appearance all contribute to a heightened awareness of death during mid-life. According to Jacques (1965), awareness of death changes people's lives in middle age, causing them to become more philosophical about their lives and to reevaluate values and priorities. In light of this developmental perspective, how does a middle-aged mother respond to the death of her adult child to AIDS?

The relationship between a middle-aged mother and an adult child is quite different from that between a mother and younger child, and differences in the grief experience can be anticipated. It may be particularly difficult to see one's offspring denied the rewards of adulthood after years of struggle for education and job security. Also, an adult-parent relationship that has been strained or has matured over time is hard to relinquish. For the mother, developmental issues related to personal losses such as retirement, widowhood or failing health affect mourning and further complicate grieving (Dane 1990).

There are different ways of coping with the death of an adult child to AIDS. Some mothers are shocked to learn that their adult sons were leading secret lives, that they engaged in life-styles difficult for the mothers to understand or accept. Others may feel either guilt about having caused their sons' homosexuality (Myers 1981–82), anger that their children were drug abusers or homosexuals, or disappointment because their children had not lived up to their expectations. Some mothers try to hide the cause of death, some feel God is punishing them and others, who were aware of their adult child's life-style, become resigned or deny the reality. Some women never come to terms with their children's deaths and lose themselves into the depths of despair and devastation. Some mothers reflect society's attitude and say "they deserved what they got." The son's lover may be blamed by the mother for her son's death, making the partner the scapegoat.

The spouse or longtime lover of the person who has died of AIDS faces many stresses after the death. When told that the loved one is dead, the typical response is numbness. The survivor feels a sense of unreality and disbelief and reports being stiff and robotlike. Although now legally a widow or an unattached lover, a woman's new status has no correspondence with her social and emotional acceptance of the role. Silverman (1981) says that only with the passage of time can the widow/lover realize that continuing to perceive herself as a wife or lover is dysfunctional in her new situation. Indeed, the need to abandon that role and the degree of reluctance to do so are critical factors in the way women cope with their bereavement.

In any conjoint relationship an equilibrium develops with respect to the roles and tasks of living, including financial matters, household tasks, emotional mutuality, sharing, dependence and sexuality. First illness and then death severely rupture this equilibrium. Sometimes the spouse, lover, mother or grandmother is unable to tolerate the stresses imposed by the death and withdraws from surviving children, grandchildren and other family members.

Because AIDS is transmitted largely through behaviors associated with homosexuality and/or drug use, it is socially unspeakable. Bereaved women who experience off-time loss hold back thoughts, emotions and feelings from virtually everyone, even clergy and mental health professionals, compounding their grief. Some fear that friends will terminate their relationships, avoid visitation or reject them if they find out about the cause of death. Others are ashamed of the behavior of their loved ones who have died from AIDS.

PSYCHOSOCIAL ASPECTS OF WOMEN SURVIVORS

Based on the authors' interviews with bereaved women and their clinical knowledge about loss and the consequences in general for survivors having lost loved ones to AIDS, certain factors can be identified in the study of women, in particular as survivors. These factors, noted also in the work of Lifton and Olson (1976), include five elements of coping similar to those discussed in the literature describing post-traumatic stress disorder: death imprint and death anxiety; death guilt; psychic numbing; nurturance conflicts; and struggle with the meaning of the loss.

Death Imprint and Death Anxiety

The first category of women's coping patterns is that of the death imprint and related death anxiety. Death imprint is when a person is plagued by memories and images of the deceased, invariably related to the last stages of deterioration and death. One can visualize this imprint as an indelible mark. For women who assumed the role of caregivers, memories were still vivid during interviews conducted several years after the deaths. The anxiety that is part of normative coping can originate from a variety of sources. Women express this in questions such as "What am I going to do now?," "How am I going to cope now that he is gone?" and, for an older widow, "Who will take care of me?"

The dissolution of a deep human relationship is a harsh and painful process that affects not only the bereaved woman but also her children and often her close relatives and friends, as illustrated in the case of Mrs. J.

Mrs. J., a fifty-six-year-old middle-aged grandmother, recalled to the therapist the memory of her second daughter's death from AIDS.

"It seemed my entire family was wiped out, even though I have three surviving children and six grandchildren. The memory of the death is very vivid, just like it happened yesterday." She continued to describe the many nights she could not sleep, waking up wondering if her grandchildren were infected with AIDS. "I know my fear is irrational, but I feel compelled to have my grandchildren tested for the virus."

Frequently people guard their anxiety around AIDS so intensely that they avoid taking actions against transmission or infection, such as having the surviving children tested. Unfortunately, many find at a later date the children are HIV-infected. In the case of Mrs. J., her grandchildren were of latency age and were born prior to their mother's drug dependency. Although she understood her fear to be irrational, to minimize her anxiety she undertook the concrete step of having the children tested. AIDS has become the enemy for many, and clinicians need to understand the sense of danger that is experienced.

Spouses like Mrs. G., a sixty-three-year-old Irish-born woman, speak to their therapists about terrifying dreams. In Mrs. G.'s case, these dreams still were recurring regularly twenty months after her husband had died from AIDS. Her husband had received an infected blood transfusion when he had undergone prostate surgery.

"In the middle of the night, I wake up sweating. This happens after the doctor in my dream tells me I have AIDS. Even though I have been tested I feel this ongoing threat." The therapist here acknowledges the reality, since a woman can become infected through sexual contact with her husband.

Coping with the death imprint and death anxiety is further illustrated in the following case of a young mother who conveyed feelings about being a parent.

Mrs. J. was a thirty-year-old woman (already known to the therapist) whose child was born and tested HIV-positive. She has intermittently seen the social worker over the past six months. Her concerns centered around her guilt over transmitting the AIDS virus to her son. The therapist acknowledged her feelings and explored the impact on her emotional well-being and on her own HIV status. After the child's birth, she initially denied that her son was born with the virus. Mrs. J. suggested that the test results were mixed up. When another blood test confirmed the diagnosis, she directed her feelings of anger at her husband, who had been a drug user several years before they were married. He had been drug-free for the past three years. "How could I have transmitted AIDS to my newborn son? I am not a prostitute or drug abuser. I would like to have more children, but I'm afraid I will kill them by giving them the virus."

As illustrated in the J. case, an infant's pending death from AIDS causes chaos, disrupts family balance and upsets the operational structure of the family. Although the initial shock, anger and chaos are felt, infected mothers like Mrs. J. have to cope with their own medical and psychosocial needs and their basic care as they are pummeled by continuous anxiety, pain, guilt and depression, all signs of grief. Ongoing counseling helped Mrs. J. care for her child until his death at nineteen months. She is presently in treatment recovering from his death and receiving medical treatment (AZT) for her illness. Some small signs of hope are beginning to emerge.

We all use denial as a defense against the fear that death evokes. Fear of death may be synonymous with fear of pain, separation or loss of self. Denial as a defense against death anxiety is believed by many to be a characteristic response in our society (Dumont & Foss 1972). Women, however, are reportedly more likely than men to contract AIDS heterosexually with high-risk partners who are intravenous drug users or bisexual (Freidland & Klein 1987). Women may unknowingly be sexually involved with HIV-infected intravenous drug-abusing partners. Or, afraid of losing their companion they may be aware of the partner's high-risk behaviors yet deny the risk themselves or the existence of the behaviors.

Clinicians need to acknowledge that some women are unaware of the unsafe sexual behavior of their mate, and that in some cultural contexts, a woman's acquiescence to sex on demand is both expected and enforced. For many women "just saying no" to sex or to unprotected sex has turned into a prescription for abandonment, battering and other forms of abuse (Bacon 1987). Among the women who are most affected by AIDS, the fact that they are still in situations of unequal power means that they now face additional obstacles to mourning.

One of the most common reactions to trauma such as an infant's death or imminent death from AIDS is a drastically heightened sense of vulnerability. A woman's previous illusions of invulnerability are suddenly shattered. Not only is this feeling of vulnerability unfamiliar, it also is accompanied by other symptoms of psychological distress. Women, like men, experience a loss of control when facing death. Although they are barely coping with or recovering from earlier blows from the illness of their loved ones, death introduces a staggering set of new conditions. Studies on depression show that the main precipitating cause of depression is not grief itself but the hopelessness that precedes the grief. Perceived vulnerability causes one to feel susceptible to future negative outcomes and unprotected from danger or misfortune.

Death-related anxiety continues to plague women in the AIDS environment, to the point of contagion. Women are not only haunted by the death of their husband, son, child or partner, but also are often threatened by the stigma and discrimination stemming from the unacceptable forms the death has taken, and feel vulnerable to the inner and outer environment.

The hopelessness of women who are infected and/or have lost their children to death from AIDS can evoke a hopelessness in the clinician (see Chapter 9). The therapeutic task and challenge for the therapist is to infuse hope while helping women find sufficient strength to cope with their grief. To the extent that the same strengths and intrapsychic processes become parallel and interactive in the professional relationship, a pattern of mutual trust, strength and hope is established, which generates nurturance and a more positive attitude.

Death Guilt

Death guilt refers to women survivors experiencing painful self-condemnation over being alive while their loved one has died. For some, this feeling will plague them until their own death. In certain situations, women express an irrational notion that they could or should have done something to save their loved one. One older mother we interviewed was preoccupied with memories of her failure to save her son from the activities and outcome of his drug use. This feeling is profound among both younger and older mothers. Death guilt is reflected in the preoccupation of women with fending off a sense of guilt and responsibility for the unacceptable death of their loved one.

Death guilt is perhaps most vivid in recurrent dreams. Some of these dreams include the reappearance of the deceased, either in everyday situations or in reunion fantasies. One dream, related by a woman who was a long-time companion of an IV drug user, involved the reliving of her partner's grotesque death, which she had witnessed. The dream reflected her perception of herself as vulnerable and helpless. Mothers, too, feel responsible for and are inconsolable over their infant's death. In therapy, they describe dreams of violence toward themselves and express feeling helpless and guilty for not protecting their child from death.

The following case illustrates the stresses women experience after the death of their loved ones:

Mrs. R., a year after her son's death, came to the Mother's Support Group with one of her acquaintances from the neighborhood. Mrs. R. was very quiet for four meetings, although the therapist felt she was listening and nonverbally acknowledging what was said. The seven other mothers in the group were very verbal, and the group conveyed a sense of caring and understanding. The therapist recognized that Mrs. R. would participate when she was ready, so neither she nor the group members put any pressure on her. Some members would ask her a question every now and then, to which she gave short answers.

At the fifth session, one mother spoke at length about how she had done all she could for her son before he had died. Although she was sad about his illness and death, she felt no guilt. Mrs. R.'s face mirrored all the emotions she was experiencing, and finally she began to talk about her son and how she was coping with his death.

"When Jose came around for Easter dinner, I knew that something was wrong. I did not see him for about a year or so, although we talked on the phone several times. He was much thinner than he had ever been, walked slowly and bumped into furniture as he moved around the apartment. Nothing was said. All four of his siblings, their spouses, and children were there. Jose's godmother had made a special effort to join us for this event. Between the eating and drinking, talking about politics in Puerto Rico and singing songs we have loved for years, we had one of the best times the family had had in a long time.

"Jose, very unlike him, stayed for a long time and seemed reluctant to leave. Several times I caught him looking at me, as if he wanted to tell me something, but the opportunity for us to be alone never seemed to arise. When he got ready to leave there was a lot of commotion as I tried to get packages of food for others to take with them. This is a family custom, and the children always talk about how good it is to have leftovers for a meal the next day. Jose didn't take any food, saying he didn't have a way to reheat the meal. What I later recall was that I didn't give him a kiss.

"That night my husband and I talked into the early morning about the get-together. When I mentioned how thin Jose looked, he tried to avoid the discussion, saying that he didn't think Jose looked any different from the time we last saw him. We had heard that Jose had been doing drugs, but none of the children wanted to tell me any details, knowing how much I disapprove of drugs. In my heart, I knew about Jose's drug use, but I could not admit it to myself. As you can imagine, the idea of his having AIDS never entered my mind, although I heard about it on the Spanish radio station.

"Four weeks later, a social worker called me from the hospital. I did not want to talk to the worker, but spent most of the month at Jose's bedside, watching him lose consciousness, not know who I was and finally die." Mrs. R. began to sob and said she cried at the funeral and has continued for the past year and a half. "The ideas which keep going around in my head is why did it have to happen to Jose, my youngest. I wish I could take his place. Children are not supposed to die before their parents. I had so many hopes for him. He was so talented. All my life I sacrificed my time, my interests and my life for him. It wasn't possible to make the ultimate sacrifice for him, although God knows I would have done so willingly."

The group remained quiet, and the therapist respected the silence. One mother reached over to Mrs. R. and comforted her with a hug and said she went through a similar situation with her daughter. The therapist conveyed the struggle to experience anger at being abandoned by their loved ones. The worker helped Mrs. R. express her justifiable anger and guilt for not being able to protect her son from death. She helped her consider her limitations as a mother rather than blaming herself. The worker helped her understand that she was punishing herself by continuing to blame herself. The worker supported the mothers in the group for all they had accomplished with their families and in particular with their deceased adult children.

In this group the worker directed her efforts at restoring the members to their level of functioning prior to the death. Providing a sympathetic and understanding relationship, the worker actively validated the appropriateness of both Mrs. R.'s and the group members' anger at their loved ones for dying. This group, providing short-term treatment, helped the members talk to each other about how they could feel less hopeless and work to improve their lives with the recognition of the loss and feelings of anger and disappointment.

Women survivors who outlive their adult children, like survivors in general, are never quite able to forgive themselves for having survived. Another side of them, however, experiences relief and gratitude that it was they who had the good fortune to survive in contrast to the fate of the deceased. This is a universal and all-too-human survivor reaction that, in turn, intensifies guilt. Since the emotion is so painful, the sense of guilt may be suppressed and covered by other emotions or behavior patterns, such as rage or apathy.

Psychic Numbing

Psychic numbing is a diminished capacity for feeling all kinds of emotions. The numbing results in various forms of apathy, withdrawal, depression and overall constriction in living. Psychic numbing is perhaps the most universal response to trauma. This syndrome is an extension of the stunned state experienced at the time of the death. That state was a defense against feeling the full impact of the overwhelming death immersion. The numbing persists when women need to defend themselves against the kinds of death anxiety and death guilt discussed earlier.

Numbing is an aspect of persistent grief, of the "half-life" defined by loss and guilt, close, at times, to an almost literal identification with the dead. One mother said to her therapist: "I feel dead now, I have no energy. I sit down and I feel numb. The only thing that gets me going is Ralph, my eight-year-old grandson. I have been caring for him the past year since his mother and then, three months later, his father died." Some women, like Mrs. O., are unable or do not have the opportunity to express their grief adequately. When the therapist first saw Mrs. O. she only talked about her daughter's death and did not mention the death of her son-in-law. Only after a more detailed exploration of the family constellation did this information surface. It became apparent that there was tremendous pain and anger associated with their deaths, but that the suppressed grief and numbing were the initial ways of coping.

For women who have lost a loved one to AIDS, this death may be just one in a series of deaths that some families, particularly in urban environments, will experience. One woman in the support group discussed earlier described having participated in six funerals of family and friends in her neighborhood in the last five months. For many women, the crisis of one death will not be resolved before another one occurs. The inability to mobilize the emotional resources needed to deal with another trauma may result in numbing and unresolved grief.

Some women describe being uninterested in seeing family members and friends or going to church or social gatherings. Even in intimate relationships the capacity of women survivors for both emotional and physical feelings tends to be greatly diminished. Women's withdrawal may be accompanied by a wide variety of psychosomatic symptoms, such as general fatigue, loss of appetite, gastrointestinal difficulties, aches and pains and dysfunction that can involve just about any organ system. One mother in the group, whose only son, a hemophiliac, had died said: "I want to be left alone. My life has been destroyed. I left my husband because he was pressuring me to get on with my life, go to work, meet with friends." Senses of abandonment and withdrawal tend to reinforce one another. Women in the group who were mothers of homosexual men referred to the death of their sons as "the end of time" or "the end of everything," and stated that "no one who does not go through this could ever really understand our experience."

Clinicians cannot underestimate the grief or the stigma associated with AIDS. Loss of enthusiasm for life has to be acknowledged. Searching for the meaning of the tragic death is helpful for some mothers, and provides a temporary way to cope. The support group described earlier gave the mothers the sense of an anchor, and although what was meaningful to them was gone, they developed a feeling of safety with each other.

Clinicians need to attend to both under- and over-activity, both of which are expressions of avoidance of feelings. Working with the denial in a benign, supportive way seems to be more helpful to the client in reducing the numbing. Monitoring the fear of attachment to the worker is helpful, as is acknowledging the difficulties in tolerating any interpersonal demands. Ongoing supportive contact through individual or group treatment seems to provide a more adaptive way of coping. As survivors are allowed to grieve at their own pace in their own way, the emotional bond is gradually dissolved and new relationships are formed. Support may also be needed from the clinician to encourage women to use healthy rather than destructive coping mechanisms.

Other aspects of numbing are memory lapses, general sluggishness, unresponsiveness, and confusion about details about the passage of time. Memory lapses, as several mothers made clear, tend to be associated with the death: "I can remember things before my daughters were diagnosed with AIDS, then I can recall the past year or months since their deaths."

Numbing is closely related to the psychological defense of denial; women say again and again, "It's hard to believe all this happened." Numbing and denial are sustained because of the survivor's inability to confront or work through the death. Feelings stay muted, psychological pain remains silent and life experience in general is drastically reduced.

Nurturance Conflicts

Much of women's lives centers on their nurturing roles as mother, lover and caretaker. To be robbed of these roles is itself a conflict. As many women reach out for human love, support and companionship after their loved ones' deaths, an equal number feel unable to accept the affection or nurturing that may be offered to them. While many women have been able to help each other, there have also been instances of breakdown and suspiciousness of the closest human bonds.

An older mother whose son had died of AIDS expressed her marriage as being on hold:

We rarely have sexual relationships or sleep in the same room. I have a great deal of anger toward my husband for not visiting our son when he was ill. He says he grieves, and hurts in his way, but I don't think he cared. . . . It hurts me to see him in pain, but there is nothing I can do, he had his chance.

This mother further reveals that she must expend considerable energy to contain her rage, saying she is afraid she would be unable to maintain control. Women, like all survivors, need the support that comes from family closeness, but they also feel a strong resentment and fear when they do get together with family members. Many times, women express their anger and jealousy at their friends whose children are alive. They feel they can not help but express their resentment in the presence of these friends. The inability to find a satisfying outlet or target tends to leave these women with no choice but to suppress their anger and maintain their continuous grief.

One woman recognized that her anger was a painful burden and responded to another mother, who encouraged her to join a mother's support group, that she would rather seek individual treatment. The need for individual treatment is illustrated in the following case of Mrs. S., who reveals how her rage and grief were "on hold" for one year before she entered therapy.

Mrs. S. is a thirty-six-year-old African-American nurse, mother of two pre-adolescent children. Her husband died of AIDS one year ago. She does not know how she handled herself this past year but feels enraged and fears she will not be able to control her anger. She begins by telling the therapist of the onset of her husband's illness as a way of becoming in control of her situation. Her husband Jim was thirty-nine years old, and worked as a successful accountant. She insisted that he see a doctor after several months of his complaining of a mild case of diarrhea and a persistent cough, which he considered to be a mild cold. The internist admitted Jim to the hospital for tests due to his difficulty with breathing.

Mrs. S. recalled Jim's rapid deterioration and her concern, which led her to pressure the doctor for more details. A week after admission, the doctor told Jim that he tested positive for HIV. He insisted on having some time to think about this before he and the doctor, jointly, shared the news with Mrs. S.

"Because of my profession and natural interest in keeping up with developments in the medical field, I read a great deal about AIDS. I was fully aware of the risk groups, the methods of transmission and the public stigma against the disease. I developed several educational forums about AIDS for the teachers, students and parents at the high school where I work. This all raced through my head when I was told about my husband's diagnosis. I was shocked and speechless. I recall forcing myself to listen to the doctor's comments and even asked some questions. I am presently at a loss to recall what the comments and questions were. I remember reaching out to hold Jim's hand and telling him that things will be all right and we will fight this together. We had a solid marriage and close relationship with our families.

"Jim became less and less communicative following our discussion with the doctor. I tried to draw him out and keep him interested in what was happening outside the hospital, with the children and their school activities, and with our mutual friends. Unfortunately, because of the children's ages—less than twelve years of age—they were not permitted to visit him in the hospital. Periodically, Jim would seem to perk up and participate in discussions of our finances.

"I continued to visit Jim daily and tried to tell myself that he would improve and before long would be home, and our lives would revert to its previous regularity. I was surprised when I got an urgent call from the hospital informing me that Jim had taken a turn for the worse. I dropped everything and rushed to see him, taking a brief pause to call his parents and two brothers. I arrived in time to have a brief chat with Jim during which he apologized for causing me and the family any pain and discomfort. He told me that he had engaged in some homosexual encounters during the last three years, but he wanted me to know that he had not loved me or the children any less. It was something he slipped into out of curiosity, not realizing it would mean death. As we talked, Jim slipped into a coma, and within the hour was dead. I was incoherent and numb when Jim's relatives arrived. They began to make plans for telling the children and other family members about his sudden death.

"Jim's brother made funeral arrangements and told the children about their father's death. I was numb throughout and his brother helped me make it through the first few days. In contrast to the way I was when Jim was hospitalized, I would stare in space and cry for hours. A week after Jim was buried, his brother and sister-in-law took the two children to spend some time with them, and I went to my parents, who live close to my two sisters.

"I did not tell my family or Jim's about the last conversation I had with him before his death. Rather I began to be more withdrawn and refused to acknowledge the expression of condolences and offers of help from family and friends. I recall spending a great deal of time alone, driving to lonely spots where I would try to think about my life with Jim. I began to feel that it was a sham, a complete lie and our marriage was meaningless. I should have known about Jim's homosexuality, recalling the many times he wished to remain in the city while the children and I went to visit his family for extended weekends or during the summer. I thought about the desk drawer which he had always kept locked, and in which I had found several gay-oriented magazines and addresses of gay meeting places. It was finding those magazines that made me feel desperate and discuss it with my sister. She listened to my difficulties and suggested it may be helpful to talk to the therapist that her friend recommended."

The worker accepted Mrs. S.'s assessment of her marital situation and her current rage at her deceased husband. She helped her express her fears of being alone and the negative effects of her husband's secretive homosexual behavior. Over the ensuing year, the worker helped Mrs. S. to become less guilty about not being emotionally available to Jim so that he sought love in men. She helped Mrs. S. reflect on the strengths of the marriage and accept that Jim's sexual behavior stemmed from his desire and not something lacking in his wife. Mrs. S. used the weekly sessions to sort out her feelings about Jim and to correct some perceptions that might be distorted. Concurrently, the worker helped Mrs. S. think through her role as a widow and single parent and become involved again in activities that would give her pleasure.

Given the possibility of transmission, the worker supported and encouraged Mrs. S. to get tested, and helped her work through her realistic fears and concerns that she would test positive. The therapist further explored ways of telling the children about the cause of their father's death and supported Mrs. S.'s wish to have her children receive therapy. Mrs. S. discussed the situation with the school psychologist and he offered the children an opportunity to participate in a group he was co-leading at the school. After two years Mrs. S. felt good about herself, but fearful of one-to-one relationships with men. She felt this was the next area to work on, to learn new ways of approaching men without being suspicious of their betrayal. She continued to monitor her negative HIV status.

Women differ in the length of time necessary to "let go" of the deceased and reorganize their lives. Even though differences exist in the mourning, there is no shortcut or escape from the emotions or energy required to reach resolution. Reintegration and comfort are attained through the support and strength of family, friends, acquaintances and, for some, thoughts of reincarnation. A grandmother felt she gained her solace through God and felt she could cry out her rage with the Lord. Some women whom we interviewed coped with the death of their loved ones by turning to religion or using a religious interpretation to comprehend what had happened. Initial responses to the death were a loss of faith, anger and sometimes hatred for a God who allowed this to happen. Some mothers who blamed God and held him responsible indicated that they felt no shame for holding these sentiments and that it felt good to hold someone responsible.

Faith and religion were eventually rekindled in the minds of grandmothers and older mothers whose adult children had died from AIDS as the only logical and satisfactory explanation for what had happened. For many, simply thinking or saying "It was a part of God's plan" provided an effective way of dealing with the loss and resolving the grief. As one comes to accept a religious explanation, one succeeds in counteracting the effects of preoccupation and can seek some meaning that is responsive to the resolution of grief (Knapp 1986). For some women, reaching beyond the scope of the rational world seems to be the only sensible way of coping with the death. For others, however, turning to God is, not the answer, and they find no relief from the trauma by redefining their religious commitment.

Struggle with the Meaning of Loss

Women survivors need to find a satisfactory explanation for their experience in order to be able to resolve the inner conflicts described above. Only by attributing some meaning and significance to the trauma are they able to find meaning and significance in the rest of their lives. Some women find comfort, or at least resignation, in the deep conviction that what happened was a matter of God's will or of some larger power that no mortal could influence.

Other women we interviewed did not see the situation in this way. They tended to remain confused, fixed in time, suffering the pain and guilt and experiencing the physical symptoms that unexpressed grief produces. One young mother whose infant son had died from AIDS and who was herself HIV-infected said she had no sense of direction in her life, and was waiting to die. Mrs. H., a Hispanic mother, was treated during the bereavement period following the death of her daughter, Alicia, to AIDS.

When Alicia died from AIDS, after several hospitalizations, Mrs. H. was offered an appointment by the social worker, who felt this would give Mrs. H. an opportunity to talk about her reactions to Alicia's death. Also the worker believed she could assist Mrs. H. with funeral arrangements. Mrs. H. looked bewildered at the social worker's comments, and took a few moments to ask whether the hospital would transport the body to the funeral home. The worker answered the question and encouraged Mrs. H. to talk about her feelings. Mrs. H. refused, saying she had to take care of business at home. The worker gave Mrs. H. her card and telephone number and suggested she make an appointment when she was ready.

Six months later, Mrs. H. called and inquired whether she could drop in to talk. The social worker agreed that she could and a time was arranged. Mrs. H. looked haggard and appeared thinner than the worker remembered. During her daily visits to the hospital, during Alicia's illness, Mrs. H. had appeared well dressed and in control of herself personally and emotionally.

Mrs. H. began by asking a number of questions. She wanted to know how Alicia contracted AIDS, what specific treatment she had received and whether the hospital had treated other children with the disease. The worker answered each question, and Mrs. H. nodded, saying that she remembered going over these same questions with the doctor and the worker when Alicia was in the hospital. She remembered the doctor saying that Alicia had received a blood transfusion from the paramedics at the scene of a car accident and several transfusions later in the hospital. The worker assessed her lack of recall and explored her concern and worries about neglect. She also permitted Mrs. H. to express her anger about Alicia's death and her feelings of helplessness. Mrs. H. did not respond but asked questions about several of the children that she met during her visits to the hospital. She specifically asked about Joan, who shared a room with Alicia. The worker said that Joan had died one week ago. Mrs. H. seemed quite shaken, but said nothing.

The worker inquired how things had gone since she had last seen Mrs. H. A flood of tears emerged as Mrs. H. talked about confiding in her minister at the Lutheran church she had attended for the past fifteen years. Those conversations had focused on trying to understand why Alicia had died and what comfort she could take from her religion. Her minister had been very patient and kind in his responses to her, and every now and then, she said, she felt less conflicted. She thought, however, that she had lost an essential part of her faith, and was not sure that she would regain it.

Mrs. H. recalled an event that occurred in her church about three weeks earlier. A family, parishioners of the church whom she had known for many years, and in fact, had socialized with extensively, recently returned from an extended stay in the Middle East. Mr. Johnson had been teaching in the American school there for several years but decided to return home because of the political uncertainty. Their youngest child was about the age Alicia would have been, and had not been baptized. Consequently, it had been announced for two weeks previously that she would be baptized during the regular worship service. Mrs. H. had had no reaction when she heard about the event, but found it impossible to sit through the part of the service when the youngster was being baptized. She found herself thinking that it should have been Alicia. Why is Alicia dead and not able to be as active and vibrant as the girl being baptized. Mrs. H. got up and left the service, and only after some time in the library, where she cried and did some hard thinking about the meaning of Alicia's death, was she able to return for the last part of the service.

Since that Sunday, things seemed to have gotten worse. Mrs. H. said: "I have tried these past six months to find answers to understand why Alicia died. My husband has tried to comfort me, but he too is sad. I asked him to come with me today, but he does not want to talk to anyone except me. I am worried because I am neglecting my responsibilities as wife and mother to my two remaining children."

The worker listened to Mrs. H. and felt that permitting her to recall the last six months and the feelings of pain attached to them was very cathartic. She said it was difficult to bury the pain that Mrs. H. was feeling and suggested that they meet regularly to work through the death of Alicia. Over the next eight weeks, Mrs. H. expressed her rage at the hospital and herself for not protecting her daughter. It was helpful for her to express her negative feelings, which were on hold, and to be able to tolerate her guilt and anger. Mrs. H. brought in pictures of Alicia and used them to recall happy memories that were shared by the family. The pictures were used to allow Mrs. H. to grieve her loss. Around the end of the first year in therapy, Mrs. H. showed the therapist pictures of her two surviving children, Paul and Scott. She used the worker's support and verbalized her concern for her husband and children. Mrs. H. began this session by saying, "I have two beautiful sons and a husband that loves me, I can't sit around and mope now that Alicia's dead. Life will not be the same, as a part of me is gone but a part of me remains." Although expressing feelings of ambivalence, Mrs. H. redefined her child's death by casting it in positive terms as a release from suffering. She told the worker that every day she prays to God and to her deceased mother, who she believes is with Alicia in heaven, to watch over her.

PICKING UP THE PIECES

During our interviews, many of the women stated that they came to understand the agony and pain in their daily lives. They came to realize there were no shortcuts to a relief from sadness, no easy way out, and that they had to make the journey alone. Remnants of "shadow grief" would remain as part of their existence. The majority of women felt that family and friends could help them face their grief and soothe the intensity of their loss. Time was often referred to as a source of hope: "In time, this will pass," or, as in the old adage, "Time will heal my wounds."

When family was unavailable there was a double hardship for some women, but they felt supported by a mental health practitioner. They felt that with professional assistance they did not have to walk alone in the wilderness of their intense emotions. Clinicians became sounding boards, permitting women to open up and verbalize their feelings and reactions, while being fully understood and accepted for who they were.

Some clinicians have used rituals to promote healing. Transforming a familiar ritual or creating a new ritual is a powerful intervention in healing, because a survivor can tailor the ritual to her individual experiences and needs. Healing is not a linear process, but a circular working and reworking. The rituals described by some clinicians show that they serve different functions and can be effective at different stages of healing. For example, a birthday celebration can help to commemorate the event, while photographs are used to facilitate the process of reminiscing or to help break the silence around the taboo of AIDS. Through rituals and creative acts, women survivors are able to relive the wonderful and painful memories and affirm that they are now strong enough to go on. Clinicians have observed the similarities between psychotherapy and creative acts and suggest that therapy itself can function as a ritual process for women.

While rituals can focus on a specific stage of healing, they are often most effective if they explicitly affirm the developmental tasks and healing stages mastered previously by the woman, and also initiate goals for the future. Individual, interpersonal and communal levels are vehicles for healing and may be important for a woman survivor.

Interpersonal contact is important for breaking through the feelings of isolation, shame and secrecy caused by a death from AIDS. Rituals can provide such interpersonal contact if they incorporate family, friends and significant others who have a history with the deceased. A woman may need to be encouraged to reach out to others as well as to strengthen her relationships to facilitate her grief.

SUPPORT GROUPS

Peer support groups, according to Levy (1979), are composed of relatively small numbers of people with common problems who meet regularly to discuss their difficulties and ways of dealing with them. These groups can be led by mental health professionals or can be self-help groups. Indeed, such groups frequently stress experiential rather than professional knowledge, often operating on the assumption that people who have endured some problem are the best experts on how to cope with it. What these groups primarily offer to survivors is the opportunity to meet and talk with other survivors, in this case, women. To the extent that AIDS survivorship prompts intense, negative feelings, women may be particularly inclined to wonder about the appropriateness of their emotional reactions. People under stress need to know that they are responding in an appropriate and normal way.

For most women, a peer self-help group that they found or join is the ideal support mechanism to help them survive the ordeal and begin the healing process. Bereaved survivors may frequently find that those around them are not very helpful in normalizing and validating their feelings. While friends and relatives may occasionally communicate to women that their sadness is normal and appropriate, these well-meaning people are likely to attempt to reduce the survivors' distress by focusing on tasks these grievers should undertake. Although significant others are trying to be helpful when they encourage the bereaved woman not to dwell on her sorrow, or to regard her problems as not so bad, since she has other surviving children, they are also implying that the person is more upset than she should be.

Barrett (1978) and Videka-Sherman (1982) concur that contact with other people sharing the same experiences does not lead survivors to see their lives as any less painful or tragic, but it does help them to see their suffering as more meaningful and therefore bearable. The realization that they are not alone, and above all, that they can help others precisely because they share their problems (Coates, Renzaglia & Embree 1983), may give survivors a sense of dignity, belonging and purpose that they would not have felt without the group experience. When women survivors remind one another that things could get worse, it may prompt more effective cognitive and behavioral preparation for later problems, even if it also produces immediate emotional distress. Finally, women as survivors may join together in the type of collective action that could ultimately prove most effective in solving their problems and quelling their grief.

In order to maximize positive outcomes in support groups, it is necessary to identify the important functions such groups serve for members. While it may be difficult for support groups to meet some of the womens' needs without thwarting others, it is not necessarily impossible. For example, the widows of longer standing in a study of a bereavement group by Vachon et al. (1980) may have been in an ideal position to provide both validation and hope to the more recent widows they met with, by emphasizing their own immediate negative reaction ("I was totally devastated at first") and their gradual recovery ("but after some time, I began to feel better"). Similarly, women who are long-term survivors of loved ones who have died from AIDS can help the newly bereaved. In professionally facilitated groups, fellow survivors may provide a sense of connectedness and meaning, while the therapist-facilitator can counteract the depressing implications of women belonging to a tragic and stigmatized outcast minority.

IMPLICATIONS FOR PRACTITIONERS

In spite of the explosion of literature on the subject of AIDS in general, relatively little is written on women as survivors. The role of grief in the lives of women, especially in AIDS epicenters, has been grossly neglected. It is common for women to endure multiple bereavements due to the death of a spouse, long-term companion, child, grandchildren and friends, and some have to confront the prospect of their own death. The potential for psychological distress is formidable.

Most women will handle their losses in their own way and will work through the entire process without experiencing an emotional problem. They will find their place among the 85% who manage without outside help (Ramsay & Noorbergen 1981). Knowing, however, that bereaved women, like other grievers, are vulnerable after the death of a loved one, the key to preventing serious physical or phychological problems is to provide services that respond to the specific needs and differences of the underserved population of women who have lost loved ones to AIDS.

AIDS has given rise to a new generation of psychological problems at each of the key landmarks over the course of the illness. Death, as experienced by women, is no exception. The complexity of emotional and behavioral symptoms of grief women experience includes profound sadness, guilt, numbing and withdrawal, and for some an increased alcohol and drug use, consistent with survivors of catastrophes and traumas. Such difficulties require recognition and response from the professional community.

The implications for clinical interventions are clear. Most vulnerable people, indeed all of us, are sustained in the community through membership in informal social networks. Awareness that significant caring is going on all around us in informal social networks is a first step. When women are bereft of support, a proactive practice is required. Mental health professionals already have a wide repertoire of theoretical models and clinical techniques with which to meet the challenges. The harsh idiosyncrasies that a woman experiences after a loved one's death from AIDS demands new levels of flexibility and personal insight on the part of mental health workers, and an extensive community outreach in the development of effective services.

Traditional approaches to treatment using individual work can be appropriate for many women, but the best approach, according to women and practitioners working with this bereaved population, involves participation in support groups. Learning coping skills through participation has been especially beneficial. It is important that women survivors incorporate some interpersonal connections in their healing processes through group or individual therapy, communal rituals or other means. The overlap between psychological symptoms caused by emotional reactions to AIDS deaths and those stemming from society's stigma requires an approach that considers the complexity of this type of bereavement.

CHAPTER 6

Intervening with Families of Homosexual and Bisexual Men

Homosexual and bisexual men, regardless of their ethnicity, culture or racial identity, are members of a family. In their family of origin they are sons, brothers, grandsons, cousins and nephews. In their family of procreation, bisexual men are fathers and husbands. When they are defined only in terms of their sexual preferences, their membership and participation in families are likely to be forgotten or overlooked and our perspective about them likely to be informed by stereotypes.

The family is known as the socializing agent through which the individual (primarily during childhood) learns how to interact with other people. Zastrow and Krist-Ashman (1987) state: "The (socialization) process involves the acquisition of language, values, etiquette, rules, behaviors, and all the subtle, complex bits of information necessary to get along and thrive in a particular society" (108).

Since our society values heterosexuality, it can be assumed that most families socialize their male members to prefer sexual relations with persons of the opposite gender as their dominant approach to sexual expression. The family and the individual both have an impact on and significance for each other. This impact and significance has to be considered in any discussion of issues related to death and bereavement.

There has been relatively little research on the survivors of homosexual men who have died of AIDS, and even less on the responses of surviving families where the husband was bisexual. The plight of these family survivors is easily overlooked by mental health professionals. Figley (1985) states that survivors do not wear a sign identifying themselves, though they are not difficult to spot—they are often the least prepared to cope with life challenges, yet least likely to seek assistance.

As the disease spreads among the larger population, there are not only homosexuals who die from AIDS, but an increasing number of bisexuals who are seropositive and will eventually contract AIDS. It is a difficult task for any clinician to review the plight of all family survivors of these men. Yet the lack of attention to family survivors of homosexual and bisexual men is unfortunate. The enormity of multiple deaths and resultant trauma is extraordinary, and acknowledgment of the psychological stresses that families experience is essential.

AIDS is (at least for now) a terminal illness, and as yet the health care system has only offered some palliatives, but no cure. The psychological consequences of the disease daily confront survivors who cope with multiple stressors stemming from the loss of their loved ones and, for some partners, uncertainty about whether they face the same illness.

Families usually play a significant role as death becomes a reality, whether the loved one dies at home or in the hospital. Families usually mobilize themselves to the tasks at hand, such as making the necessary funeral arrangements. The post-death mourning phase has unique features for families of homosexual and bisexual men, and mental health professionals working with this population need to be attendant to these unique factors to help these families through the stages of grief and to enable them to avoid a pattern of enmeshment around fear, secrecy and shame.

This chapter will discuss the characteristics of AIDS and the impact of the illness on families of homosexual and bisexual men for whom professional intervention should be considered. The following areas will be discussed: (l) the emotional effects on families; (2) patterns of communication; (3) multiple stressful events; and (4) the role of support groups. To elucidate the stresses that families experience as they grieve the death of their members, case examples will illustrate methods of coping with death from AIDS. Unlike cancer or other life-threatening illnesses, AIDS suggests a life-style that carries with it a social stigma, which isolates the family from the community comfort and support that is readily available to other families. The clinician who works with family survivors must be alert to the differences between survivors of persons who have died of AIDS and survivors of those who have died of other causes, yet must also consider the similarities of social and emotional exile imposed on all mourners.

It is evident that families will experience conflict, disruption, disintegration, alienation and social isolation. These families must be regarded at high risk because of the inevitable feelings of shame and guilt, and possible alienation from neighbors, friends and extended family. AIDS is a family problem that transcends illness and death. It is uniquely one that causes families to feel they have failed and have a "skeleton in the closet."

EMOTIONAL EFFECTS ON FAMILIES

Families who have lost someone to the ravages of AIDS experience multifaceted repercussions. AIDS is a catalyst that can divide a family. Given the isolation many homosexual and some bisexual men experience in relation to their families, the question of what effects the death of a son, husband or father have on a family becomes a focus of concern. Families of gay men with AIDS are less available to them than are families of heterosexuals dealing with serious illnesses (Christ & Wiener 1985; Cleveland et al. 1988; Garrett 1988; Ryan 1988; Tiblier, Walker & Rolland 1989). Wolcott et al. (1986) found that 52% of the sample in their study of homosexual men had one or fewer family members in their current social network. Christ and Wiener (1985) found that 62% of their sample of persons with AIDS had either minimal or no contact with their families of origin. It should be noted that homosexual men have found a family support system through the gay community.

The process of building a support network to minimize emotional tension and facilitate grief work for families with a homosexual or bisexual member is not easy. Often there is tension between the family of origin, particularly one's parents and siblings; the family of procreation, one's spouse and children; and the homosexual couple. Macklin (1989) refers to this tension in her description of the "family of function." This family comprises those individuals who constitute an ongoing social and affectional intimate support network for one another, as is often apparent in situations involving gay men. Members of one's family of function provide a broad range of emotional and material support for one another, fulfilling many of the major responsibilities and roles of the traditional family. During the mourning period, whether one is discussing family of origin, procreation or function, emphasis on the impact of responsibilities, supports and tensions must be addressed by the clinician.

Tragedy and disaster often stir up opposing forces of heroics and bravery, and AIDS is no exception. Impending death can give new meaning to life. Sontag (1989) in her book, *AIDS & Its Metaphors*, states that "illness is the night side of life, a more onerous citizenship. Everyone who is born holds a dual citizenship in the Kingdom of the well and the Kingdom of the sick" (3). This can apply to those families whose experience of being involved with an ill member produces a transformation in which their love transcends their differences and the family finds great strength and cohesion (Cleveland et al. 1988; Lovejoy 1989; Tiblier, Walker & Rolland 1989).

When families acknowledge the reality of the death of the homosexual or bisexual member, intense emotions are aroused. Paradoxically, at first they may experience a transient sense of relief, sometimes with simultaneous guilt over having been so relieved. Relief is most frequently reported when the person with AIDS had manifested increasing disorientation and deterioration for a prolonged period before death, and when families had endured a lengthy emotional upheaval over the stigma of AIDS and the regime of caregiving.

Although grief work is an important aspect of every stage of dying, the death of a loved one from AIDS and its aftermath is a particularly difficult and stressful period. The central affect aroused by the death is, of course, sorrow. It is doubtful whether sorrow can be assuaged by professional intervention. However, the following factors, if understood, can assist practitioners who intervene in the complex process of mourning when families feel burdened and have lost hope.

Over the years there has been a complete lack of restraint among the press and media, churches and the clergy, politicians and professionals in all walks of life in condemning both homosexual and bisexual men with AIDS and, indirectly, their survivors. The reasons for this disapproval are as varied as those expressing it. This censure has made it extremely uncomfortable for parents, wives, siblings, children, brothers, sisters and extended family to express intense feelings of loss and anger and to grieve openly. Family members are afraid of the reactions of others. They must cope not only with the death of their loved one from AIDS but with the possible disclosure of a sexual orientation that carries a social stigma. While their hearts are burdened with shame or guilt and as they shed their tears of pain and sorrow, they do so in silence, and many remain hidden grievers.

The death of a homosexual or bisexual adult child seriously challenges the sense of parental competence and sacred obligation. "You are supposed to be able to protect your child," one mother in our interview said, "but I couldn't protect him from doing one foolish thing and that one act cost him his life. I feel like a failure." Because their sense of competence has been challenged, many parents, such as Mr. and Mrs. J., attempt to resolve the issues of competence early in the bereavement process. For these families, engagement with a clinician prior to the death fosters continuity in treatment around issues that emerge later.

Mrs. J. called to request an appointment with the social worker in the AIDS clinic when it became clear that their son's death was imminent. In her first interview, she told the worker that her major concern was her husband's steadfast refusal to allow Ben's longtime partner to visit him and his threats to exclude him and other friends from participating in the funeral. She described her sense of helplessness in the face of her husband's adamant stance and raised some minimal concerns about what she might have done to prevent Ben from leaving home.

The worker inquired about Mrs. J.'s feelings about her son's illness and the fact that he might die soon. Mrs. J. began crying as she told the worker about how promising Ben was from his earliest years of schooling through law school. She fully expected him to become a very important person and perhaps surpass his father's accomplishments as a lawyer. She described him as having an artistic flair, able to play the piano and being very good in social relationships. He had always had a good relationship with his two sisters, who have kept contact with him even while he was living in San Francisco.

She told about how sad it was to see him so ill, suffering so much pain while still trying to respond to the interests and concerns of other family members. She knew that she would miss him a great deal, because they have talked about so many different areas of life and have similar views about things. "He has been easier to talk with than my husband, at times."

The worker helped Mrs. J. to understand how she was grieving Ben's death, even though he was still alive. She reviewed the range of emotions that Mrs. J. had been feeling, her anger at this untimely death, her feelings of guilt when she thinks of things she might have done differently with Ben, and her disappointment about things that will never be, given that he would die before realizing his maximum potential. In addition, the worker provided Mrs. J. with information about AIDS and about available resources, plus information to aid her day-to-day caretaking responsibilities. The worker also provided emotional support to Mrs. J. as she faced her grief.

When Mrs. J. appeared more in control of her emotions, the worker asked whether Mr. J. would join her for the next few sessions. Mrs. J. was convinced that he would not agree to participate, but she indicated that she would ask him. The worker considered with her various ways of opening up the subject and the potential responses that Mr. J. might make. Mrs. J. left the session, after saying that she felt prepared to confront her husband and hoped that she would be able to hold her anger in check if he responded as she thought he might.

Mrs. J. called two days later to tell the worker that Ben died the previous evening. The worker expressed her condolences and repeated her invitation to Mrs. J. and her husband for a joint session. Mrs. J. agreed to meet with the worker about two days after the funeral.

Older parents of homosexual or bisexual men undergo a transient but agonizing process of self-examination and self-reproach. The family's concept of the etiology of their adult child's infection may be guilt-laden. The illness may be interpreted as God's punishment for sinfulness or, for some, viewed as God's challenge to families selected for their spiritual strengths.

Guilt for families of both homosexual and bisexual men may arise from ambivalence in the relationship. For example, if the parents did not accept the son's life-style or if the wife agreed to an open marriage, the death may be viewed as a consequence of rejection. A wife cried and said, "My feelings were intermixed over a period of three years when my husband related his affairs with men. All I could say was 'what did I do wrong?' " A father blurted out, "I felt that early prejudices and remarks were coming back to haunt me."

If the deceased person was rivalrous, negative or hostile toward the family, the survivors may have some feelings of self-recrimination. One-eighty-year old father said, "My son continued to tell us we were ignorant of homosexuality." "The entire concept of homosexuality was so foreign to me," said another mother, "that I wondered if my son could be gay and be happy. Now that he's dead I feel he will no longer be discriminated against." As parents become more informed about homosexuality, they often recognize it is possible for a homosexual son to be happy.

Awareness of a son's life-style sometimes stimulates anger toward the surviving lover, particularly if the lover is, or is thought to be, HIV-positive— perhaps having transmitted the disease to the person who died. Displaced anger may exert a destructive influence on meaningful and necessary relationships. Family members who acknowledge their anger, recognize its displacement and discharge it through nondestructive channels free themselves to utilize other family members and their son's lover for sources of emotional support. Such parents respect their son's wishes, and, for example, include the lover in planning the funeral and death rituals.

The journey of social isolation is not necessarily the inevitable course for all survivors. Some families who were involved in the caregiving role feel they had some time to cope with feelings of guilt, anger and helplessness. They are knowledgeable about community resources and assistance programs and have received support from family members and health care professionals. Older parents, in particular, with the help of two organizations, Parents and Friends of Lesbians and Gays (P-FLAG) and the National Federation of Parents and Friends of Gays (P-FOG), feel supported in their struggle to accept their son's homosexuality.

Families who have sought to keep the cause of death and its circumstances a secret, however, do not obtain the customary support that grievers usually receive at the time of death. They have deprived themselves of relationships with their son's lover and/or wife and other family members to protect themselves from what is perceived as an unwelcome reality. Many live with anger and guilt, compounded by the fear that they will be discovered. The longer families cling to their long-held fantasies of marriage, family and a heterosexual life-style for their children, the longer the mourning process takes and the more difficult it is to accept the death.

Fear of family and friends finding out the cause of death, especially for wives of husbands who have died of AIDS, has prompted many to protect themselves and their children with a web of secrecy. Avoidant reactions of others can heighten distress and leave survivors feeling shunned, vulnerable and isolated from the very persons who had previously been a dependable source of support. Harboring the secret and refusing to communicate often amplifies these feelings and extends the grief over a much longer period of time. The longer the silence continues, the more likely that grief resolution will be hampered. Imposed isolation, as reflected below in the case of Mr. and Mrs. J., seems to be a combination of distancing by the family and significant others and censuring by society.

As Mr. J. arrived for the first joint session with his wife following the death of their son, he was visibly angry. The worker noted his emotional reactions and began to explore this with him. Mr. J. said that he was very upset because his wife and two daughters were angry at him because of his refusal to allow Ben's friends to visit him in the hospital and to attend the funeral. "They couldn't understand that I did not want a bunch of faggots parading around my neighborhood, and having my friends and neighbors talking about us."

The worker acknowledged his anger and his disappointment with Ben. Mr. J., fighting back tears, recalled his relief that Ben had moved away, coupled with his anger at "not having a son in my life." The session revolved around Mr. J.'s ventilating a lot of previously controlled feelings, and the worker helping him to grieve over Ben's death and old unresolved wounds. Mrs. J. cried throughout the session but indicated that she felt relieved that they were at last talking. She requested follow-up sessions, to which the worker agreed.

Mrs. J. began the second session, again expressing her pleasure regarding the work they had initiated. She commented that "for the first time this week, my husband and I began to really talk about Ben." Mr. J. responded, saying that "Ben's life-style has always been difficult for the family." He recalled that Ben had become aware of his sexual preference in high school and seemed determined to openly live a homosexual life-style. Ben refused to go to the prom and threatened the family that he would come out publicly. Mr. J. reported being scared that his partners in the law firm would become aware of Ben's homosexuality. "I was later concerned that our friends would also become aware of Ben's activities in the gay community and that the stigma would reflect on us. I was happy when Ben decided to relocate to San Francisco, since the move made it less likely that my colleagues and friends would hear about Ben and his activities. It also gave me a chance to be selective about what I revealed about Ben's career."

The worker acknowledged that there is a great deal of societal stigma against gays and their families. This led to fuller exploration of Mr. and Mrs. J.'s experiences with being the parents of a homosexual. They each shared secrets that they had kept from each other, from friends and from their minister. Mr. J. stated that he felt uncomfortable about telling his minister and fellow parishioners about Ben. "I still have not revealed that Ben died of AIDS." The worker explored the theme of stigma throughout the session, helping the couple to appreciate that they were not alone and to consider ways in which they might respond to others.

In subsequent sessions Mr. J. reported that he talked with one of his closest colleagues, who responded very sympathetically to his situation. "I was pleasantly surprised at the depth of understanding and empathy with which he responded."

The family bereaved by AIDS in this culture occupies a marginal social position and faces numerous taboos. The death is kept within the family system. All the family members who were linked to the deceased person in a matrix of interlocking roles must now find new roles. It is not surprising that the powerful stigma of death to AIDS creates a new family structure, with new coalitions and new boundaries. Family boundaries may become more rigid as the family interfaces with community systems and learns to keep its own counsel out of fear of being stigmatized at work, by friends, at school or at places of worship.

Dysfunctional family structures, boundaries, rituals and rules are often forms of adaptation to illness, death or pain. Dysfunctional rules, for example, not discussing the son's life-style and the associated behaviors, are observed frequently as family defense mechanisms, such as denial, isolation and secrecy. Changing the rules or promoting flexibility enables the family to move from a maladaptive response to one that promotes empowerment and recovery.

The tendency toward blaming and judging in American society is a critical barrier to empowerment of families. In the last few years, we have seen rampant blaming of persons with AIDS and their family members. Society must learn new behaviors, develop more flexible rules of acceptance and choose a response that will bring about recovery for grieved families who experience emotional suffering and psychological trauma.

PATTERNS OF COMMUNICATION

Talking about sensitive issues is never easy. With the exception of suicide, it is difficult to imagine another form of death that forces reflections on family communication to as great an extent as the death of a member from AIDS. Even the most liberal and accepting family members probably have some reservations about the relative value of the homosexual or bisexual life-style of the person who died. Families of the deceased, in particular parents, express vague guilt over their permissiveness, strictness, closeness, distance, acceptance, lack of acceptance or other qualities specific to their relationship.

Dealing with death from AIDS involves a number of complex communication issues for families of homosexual and bisexual men. Communication plays a central role in the overall resolution of grief. Communication, or lack of it, over the lifetime of the deceased person is often embedded in broader psychosocial dimensions that existed prior to the death, which now can create substantial problems that strongly affect how families cope with the death.

Family theorists suggest that during times of stress, communication can become restricted as family members try to protect themselves and others from painful feelings (Bowen 1978). Concealment of feelings is a process in which family members consciously withhold or hide emotional concerns from one another. Glaser and Strauss (1967) use the term mutual pretense to describe the phenomenon in which people have some awareness of information or feelings but pretend otherwise. Although family members hope to protect one another by concealing their feelings, the end result is that they often bear their emotional pain alone. It is ironic that family members may harbor similar feelings, which they do not share with each other.

What happens when family members conceal their feelings or restrict their communication about death to AIDS? A number of investigations have reported that closed communication can hinder family relationships. Krant and Johnston (1977-78) report that limited communication can lead to confusion within the family system. Family members with limited communication are often unsure of what other family members knew or what the deceased person told the family prior to death.

Families that communicate openly among themselves have reported more positive outcomes than families that communicate less openly. For example, Spinetta and Maloney (1978) discover that families that communicate openly report more positive coping strategies in their children. One can conclude that such families are better able to negotiate role changes within the family after death. Cohen, Dizenhuz and Winget (1977) find that family members who communicate openly with each other seem to adjust better during bereavement.

Secrecy of "Telling"

The choice of telling about the deceased person's life-style and the feelings of powerlessness in the face of stigma confront family members, resulting in loss of control. As Blumberg, Flaherty and Lewis (1980) suggest, loss of control implies a sense of dependence and lack of autonomy, and results in feelings of vulnerability. Gaining a sense of control is difficult for bereaved families of homosexual and bisexual men because of the stigma of a death from AIDS. Although significant advances have been made over the past ten years, the diagnosis and resulting death from AIDS is often regarded with more fear and as more of a threat than other deaths.

In addition to creating fear, AIDS is a disease that often involves a high degree of uncertainty regarding how a family may be perceived and accepted in the community after disclosure. AIDS is different from other illnesses such as cancer, since it is directly related to the person's behavior. Because AIDS is so frightening and unpredictable, families need interpersonal and environmental contexts that allow them to regain a sense of competence in communication, and therefore control.

The problems involved in deciding which persons can be told the truth are very real and can have tremendous negative implications. Parents, wives, children and siblings are apt to come forth with expressions of anger and ambivalence about having a brother, husband, father or son die from AIDS. Deciding which friends to tell the truth and which ones to lie to or be vague with also poses concern. When families lie, suggesting for example that their relative died of cancer, they do not get the support they need. Telling the truth entails revealing secrets of a sexual identity and life-style that is extremely threatening to a family's position in the community.

In situations where a man has been living a dual life, there has usually been some degree of accommodation in the family dynamics. This may be conscious, but most often it is unconscious, or at least out of awareness. Some men have been emotionally unavailable to their wives and children all along and, as a result, the discovery of their situation is less emotionally intense for their family. Such families may, however, get in touch with feelings of neglect and intense anger (Rodway & Wright,1988). The ability of families to work through this massive assault on their roles and family systems is drastically curtailed unless they can communicate with each other and have the support of extended family and friends.

Children

Children are often bewildered by the isolation and secrecy surrounding death from AIDS (this is discussed more fully in Chapter 4). It is hard to grieve when one cannot openly discuss the cause of death. Closely related to the family's need to maintain a sense of control is the need to seek information. For children the acquisition of information is a primary means of regaining a sense of understanding of their father's death. Information is generally beneficial, because it helps them feel that their responses to the trauma of the death are reasonable and normal.

The wife of a person with AIDS has to work through her understanding of the husband's sexual practices as well as her feelings of anger and the grim realities of her own life if she tests positive for AIDS. In attempting to meet the informational needs of the children, mothers are forced to confront questions such as: "How much information do the children want?" "What kind of information is most important to them?" and "From whom do they want the information?" Information is empowering and builds hope by freeing children from the anxiety and fear related to the uncertainties of surviving a father's death to AIDS.

Adults frequently attempt to explain death to children in euphemistic terms, in the conviction that it will be easier for youngsters to understand and accept. In the case of AIDS, explaining death in terms of morality ("God took Daddy to heaven") or in simplistic terms ("Daddy has gone to sleep") may lead a young child to develop irrational fears having to do with going to sleep and never waking up, or feeling that her/his father was "bad" and punished with an untimely death.

Even as they struggle with their own grief, it is helpful for adults to consider the child's level of development as they seek to explain death or aid in the child's grief work. Preschool children can appreciate an explanation that involves the body not being able to continue working. Adolescents, on the other hand, who have a fairly well-developed concept of death, may need help with their sense of vulnerability, with conflicts about moving away from the family and developing a sense of autonomy. They are likely to have some information about AIDS, methods of contracting the disease and the stigma associated with it. It is critical that adults not exacerbate their conflicts by being reluctant to talk about the disease and death or by expressing their unresolved conflicts about the deceased person.

Disclosure of feelings plays a pivotal role in helping individuals adjust to the crisis of death. Families have different needs for disclosure at various stages of mourning. Although some evidence of healing is observed when individuals engage in honest and open communication, disclosure outside the family is often a problem because other people may avoid talking with them or may express retaliation in various ways. Awareness of the deleterious consequences of disclosure can help set the pace for what and how much families want to disclose about their experience. Teenagers have expressed anger about the perceived preferential treatment they received from teachers and family members. They also report that their friends stayed away from them after hearing their father's cause of death and seemed to be afraid of catching the disease.

Concerns about concealing feelings and coping with feelings of helplessness affect the ability of family members to mourn openly. Survivors have shared many rich personal accounts of their experiences and difficulties in communicating both within and outside the family. For surviving family members caught in double-bind situations such as death to AIDS, supportive communication eases the distress and enhances coping.

Siblings

Most family members experience feelings of guilt over the death of a loved one, and siblings are no exception. Many adult siblings whom we interviewed experienced guilt for being alive when their brother died, for having been well when their brother was ill, for past disagreements with their brother over his sexual preference, for having wished their brother dead and for feeling jealous of the parent's grief over the deceased sibling. Some siblings reported feeling special when their homosexual brother left the household a number of years before his death, and felt guilty because of this.

Some siblings, in particular sisters, often assigned responsibility to themselves for events over which they had no control. Some knew of the secret life of their deceased homosexual brother and felt that they should have been more encouraging of him to come home for special family events and holidays. Others with a bisexual brother related regrets that they did not soften their parents' attitudes toward their brother and his wife, alienating the grandchildren from visits and a closer relationship with their paternal grandparents.

Guilt is not the only emotion experienced by siblings when a brother dies. Many reported having experienced intense, painful feelings surrounding the loss, and said they were unable to share their reactions with anyone. Two surviving sisters spoke of their involvement in caring for their brother prior to his death. One sister became involved after her brother's lover left, feeling overwhelmed with grief over the pending loss and his own deteriorating health. She spoke of moving in with her brother and being instrumental in having the family of origin become reunited. Prior to the death, she said, "I never heard my mother mention my brother's name or refer to him in any way." She also recalled her father becoming severely depressed and drinking heavily after her brother left the family's home. Her parents' marriage became brittle and normal frustrations snowballed into intolerable anxiety until the father's death.

Another female sibling volunteered her time at Gay Men's Health Crisis, and by attending a group for families of persons with AIDS, reached out to her brother and his lover during his ongoing bout with the illness. She related the experience of remaining with her brother overnight in the hospital one day prior to his death. She felt this gave her an opportunity for closeness and a way to console herself.

Possible reasons for women to be attached to a homosexual brother may be different patterns of socialization for women than for men, and a greater propensity among women to engage in help-seeking behaviors. No male siblings were involved in the study.

The J. family, to whom we referred above, illustrates how conflicts about the life-style of the deceased person can create friction among family members, specifically siblings.

As the therapist continued to work with Mr. and Mrs. J., they revealed that Ben's two sisters were also struggling with their grief. The worker suggested that they hold a family session.

The session began as the two daughters told that they had been very supportive of Ben's plans to relocate to San Francisco, where he had many friends and where he could meet and be with others who shared his life-style. During the years that he was away, they maintained active communication through letters and telephone calls. Jennifer said that she had visited Ben and met his lover. Both daughters stated that they had never revealed this to their parents. The worker acknowledged the burden of keeping secrets. Jennifer and Ann discussed their anger about the fact that Ben had not been able to tell the family about his illness soon after the diagnosis, fearing his father's reactions. They said that they still find it difficult to understand how their father could have been so rejecting of his only son.

Mr. J. was very defensive and claimed that he had good reasons for his feelings. He commented that when he learned about Ben's illness, he was not surprised. He revealed for the first time that while Ben lived at home, Mr. J. frequently drove by one of the local gay haunts to see if Ben's car was in the parking lot. He indicated that he had, in fact, on many occasions recognized the license plate. Both daughters and mother were appalled and angry, and accused Mr. J. of being devious. They indicated that they fully understood why Ben had not been able to trust him or be the son he really wanted.

The worker supported how difficult it was for all of them to keep secrets from each other and wondered what it was like now to hear how involved they were with Ben. Throughout the remainder of the session, the worker attended to open communication within the family. Acting in the role of mediator, the worker explored the family's fear about stigma, secrecy and guilt.

Jennifer expressed her anger about Ben's lover not being able to see him in the hospital or attend the funeral. She wondered if he could come to visit, and Mr. J. indicated that he needed a little time before he could have Paul visit their home. They agreed to use the next few sessions to consider what Paul's visit meant and its implications for them as a family.

The AIDS crisis may serve as a growth experience in that to maintain a marriage or family ties in the face of such a tragedy, families have to develop more effective communication. Some families experience personal growth, especially in the area of interpersonal communication, following the death of their loved one.

MULTIPLE STRESSFUL EVENTS

The discussion throughout this book has reflected the multifaceted nature of grief, bereavement and mourning. While AIDS survivors are confronted with their grief work, they nevertheless have to cope with aspects of daily life (the responsibility for which may be assumed by significant others), frequently with financial and social concerns, and with shifts in their social status. Grief involves emotional, behavioral and spiritual processes, each with their inherent demands and stresses. Dershimer (1990) observes that grief "includes significant changes in the behavior, thoughts, attitudes, and in the religious and spiritual life of the bereaved. Relationships change, new friendships are formed with those who understand and are comfortable with grief, and existing friendships change in character and mourning" (17).

Mourning may not be a single process, but may entail multiple processes. Death is always difficult to confront, and uncertainty looms for survivors who must come to final terms with their feelings about the life-style of the deceased person and the broader social and emotional implications of AIDS. Each family perceives the future and a place for their loved one that includes their use of talents and energies. Tremendous suffering attends the loss of hope when receiving the initial news of the diagnosis and, for some, at the same time hearing of their loved one's homosexual or bisexual life-style. For some families this awareness precipitates a challenge to their fundamental values and beliefs. Relinquishing hope and acknowledging the finality of death sets the course for grief reactions.

Acute grief is almost always present as the result of the imminent or sudden death of children, young adults and middle-aged people whose lives and living have been tragically thwarted and whose responsibilities have not been discharged or fulfilled. A death accompanied by extreme physical suffering and a disenfranchised status can also evoke acute grief with its accompanying feelings of rage and helplessness.

Families of Bisexual Men

The number of bisexual men who live a life as a husband and father and at the same time have a secret, sexually active homosexual life is difficult to ascertain. Informal reports from the gay community suggest there is a substantial group of men that fall into this category, but it is unlikely that the percentage of married men who are bisexual is high. The risk of contracting AIDS has been high for this group, since they are more likely to frequent the parks, bars and baths in a quest for anonymous sexual contact. The ramifications for wives and children are significant and complicated when their husband/father dies of AIDS. While many reactions and responses emerge at the time of diagnosis, a second trauma is activated upon the death. There are similar factors that influence the bereaved families of homosexual men, but we will identify some factors unique to the families of bisexual men.

According to Rodway and Wright (1988), for many, the diagnosis results in a dual discovery that the man has a contagious terminal disease and that he has been involved in homosexual activity. The normal reactions to the discovery that the father in the household is terminally ill are confounded. An immediate question that is raised for the spouse is her own risk of infection. To have been placed at such risk by her husband's sexual infidelity is an enormous psychological shock for most women. There may be prolonged bitterness when the wife has been unaware of her husband's extramarital affairs or activities, and she is worried that she may be infected, even though current tests are negative. In the case that the mother is infected and will die, leaving the children parentless, reorganization and preparation for custody are undertaken. The resulting anger and hurt tend to be immobilizing at a time when all of the wife's emotional resources are needed to deal with her impending loss.

Appropriate management of the children's reactions to the father's death and the mother's illness needs to be quickly addressed. Some children's fantasy and reality are interwoven. The death may be perceived as the realization of their own hostile thoughts and impulses toward the parent(s). "Is it my fault?" is therefore a paramount question. "Could it happen to me?" constitutes a question of comparable importance. Although neither question may be stated directly, children need to be reassured.

Children may interpret the mother's altered emotional state and her preoccupation as reflecting withdrawal of love and interest in them. They may feel hostile toward the surviving parent. The question of what information to share about their father's life-style must depend upon the children's stage of development. Parents can help their children by providing channels for expressing their feelings and utilizing other family members such as grandmothers, aunts and uncles to provide emotional support. Support from extended family members and clergy can help the surviving spouse and children to assimilate the reality of the death. Their support can reduce feelings of loneliness, temporarily satisfy heightened dependency needs, and afford some gratification experiences. When the extended family is not available, professional persons and support groups may play a critical substitute role.

Alterations in the life-style of the family of bisexual men result from the medical needs of the PWA as well as from the economic and emotional burden of the AIDS. The economic burden of the illness and death may extend far beyond the primary costs of medical and funeral expenses, which in themselves may be catastrophic. The family's social, recreational and educational

needs may be seriously compromised by this immense drain on family resources, and there may be a significant alteration of life-style combined with
the emotional demands of survivorship.

Families of Homosexual Men

Feelings of hurt, sadness and depression are often experienced or reex-
perienced by families as they hear the news of their son's homosexuality and
then his diagnosis of AIDS. The journey from shock to acceptance needs to
be resolved over the course of the illness in order for families to readjust and
cope with the death. Sometimes, during the course of the illness, families
of homosexual men are reconciled. Often this is at the request of the person
who is ill.

Parents of homosexual men often feel a degree of guilt and inadequacy
that they were not able to protect their child from a life-style that was
apparently responsible for his death. They also have conflicting feelings about
a child who dies before them.

Following a son's death, the mourning process may be complicated and
intensified for parents who did not accept the life-style or their son's lover.
Many times they not only share negative attitudes toward homosexuality,
but also have fears and misconceptions about AIDS. Some parents, upon
learning of their son's diagnosis of AIDS, have relocated their son to their
home and have forbidden the son's lover to have any contact. When the son
died, some lovers have not been able to attend the memorial or funeral
services.

For many parents whose sons have died of AIDS, the death separated the
deceased person from his family and created friction between the family of
origin and the family of function. A common family preoccupation is what
to tell friends and relatives if they permit their son's lover to become part of
their lives. Some families feel burdened enough without risking disapproval
or rejection from their relatives or friends, and decide to cut off contact with
their son's lover. Others find comfort in treating the lover as an extended
family member; they offer a room in their home during the illness and permit
involvement in caregiving and in planning the funeral rituals. Many parents
feel that once they have adjusted to coping with their son's life-style and
death, they can be honest with themselves, friends and neighbors and face
the disruption that would emerge from the disclosure.

Although mothers and fathers differ in their grief reactions toward the
death of their homosexual sons, it is unclear whether mothers and fathers
also differ in the length of time each takes to comes to terms with the loss.

Children of Bisexual Men

Children of a bisexual father have a difficult, doubly stressful adjustment
upon learning of the father's diagnosis and his life-style. They must juxtapose

their feelings related to his death with their feelings of shame and anger. This is compounded when they are unaware of the father's bisexuality until after his death.

Dan, a fifteen-year-old adolescent of Irish heritage, returned to school after a week's absence because of his father's death. The school social worker had been alerted by the principal that the death was from AIDS. The school took a preventive approach to problems, so that when Dan was observed to be inattentive in class and to be listless and withdrawn, the social worker arranged an appointment with him. Dan had talked with the social worker several times before, when he was concerned about his own sexual development.

The worker decided to be direct with Dan, and informed him that he was aware that his father had died recently and that families have difficulties talking to each other when they are grieving. He wondered how things were going with Dan, who immediately convulsed with tears. He told the worker that he missed his father immensely, had thought about the many things they had done together and the plans they had been making for the summer to take a camping trip. The worker acknowledged Dan's sadness and disappointment, and his feelings that life would probably never be the same again.

Dan agreed, and talked about the fact that his mother sat around for extended periods sad and crying, unable to take care of things at home. He and his two sisters frequently went hungry because his mother had not prepared dinner, and they were trying to keep the house and their clothes clean. The worker engaged Dan in discussing why his mother's grief was so extensive. Dan cried throughout the interview, repeatedly expressing his wish that things would be as they were when his father was alive and well. The worker talked about this being a safe place for Dan to come and express and talk about his feelings. He talked with Dan about ways he might use to keep up with his school work and helped him to use other resources in the school as a way of coping.

In the second interview, Dan was visibly uncomfortable and avoided looking directly at Mr. Franklin, the social worker. They talked routinely about how things were going since they talked last week and whether Dan felt there was any improvement at home. Dan agreed that they were somewhat better, and then began talking about his father's death and funeral. He was shocked at how his father had deteriorated and how they had tried to make him look good for the burial. Dan began to cry softly when he was asked how it was seeing his father in the coffin. He became more agitated, until he blurted out that he was still mad at his father. As the worker explored what he meant, Dan revealed that he learned that his father was bisexual during his illness and that he may have become ill because of being involved with many partners.

Dan said that he couldn't understand why his father would be interested in having sex with men and women, when he was supposed to be faithful to his wife and children. Dan indicated that he planned to be very different when he grew up. Mr. Franklin used the remainder of the session to attend to Dan's sense of vulnerability and his questions about his own sexuality. He allowed Dan to move back and forth in his comments about how angry and disappointed he was with his father, and at the same time, recalling some of the pleasant memories that he had of things they did together. Mr. Franklin talked with Dan about the anger that many people feel about someone who has died, and suggested that, with time, Dan would be able to come to grips with his feelings about his father. Mr. Franklin suggested that they might continue to talk about this and other issues that might come up in the near future.

During the subsequent seven months before the school year ended, Dan met regularly with Mr. Franklin and talked about his sadness and loneliness, his efforts to get his mother functioning again, his memories about his father and how he dealt with some of the questions and comments made by his fellow students. As the year ended, Dan indicated that he felt relieved for having talked with Mr. Franklin, and noted that he had a little better perspective about himself and his relations with his father. He mentioned that his uncle had offered to take him on the camping trip that had been planned with his father, and he felt that this would help him with some of the disappointment he had been feeling.

Many teenagers, especially boys, have a difficult time because of their struggles around their own sexual identity. A clinician who works with adolescent AIDS survivors states that most attempt to maintain the secret of the cause of their father's death and fear deleterious consequences of disclosure. Conflicted feelings emerge when friends and teachers offer sympathy and support. At the death of a parent, separation is made worse for some children by separation from brothers and sisters. Some siblings have been split up by the parent's death, many times after a period of exceptional closeness during the parent's terminal phase of illness. Older siblings have assumed parenting roles during this time, when the mother was both caring for her husband and insulating the children for fear the diagnosis would be discovered.

Funeral Rituals

Several authors have addressed the question of how personal philosophy can affect one's way of coping with hardships. Rituals can provide meaning and value to the continued existence of the survivor, and memorialize memories of the deceased. Jourard (1971) suggests that when people find hope, meaning, purpose and value in existence, they become inspired, which, in turn, makes them more effective and more capable of combating grief. Rituals can be helpful during the mourning period and after it presumably has ended, and can be designed to help the family's healing process.

Six months after her husband's death, at a gathering of family and friends, a wife described how the death of her bisexual husband forced her to look closely at her own priorities and to reassess how she wanted to spend her time. "My priorities, pleasures and expectations began to change. I came to realize that I could have whatever aspirations I chose to have, in spite of the tragic death of my husband to AIDS." Each person, in turn, suggested how the untimely death of their friend forced them to take stock of their lives and develop creative ways to approach their everyday stresses.

Anniversaries

Anniversaries and various other times during the year--birthdays, days of deaths, holidays of various kinds—are particularly difficult for the family. They are both important times and troublesome times. These are the times that tend to keep the subdued expressions of grief alive. Newly bereaved families are still so depressed and sad at their loss that they cannot imagine being in a mood of joy and happiness. For others, looking back at past celebrations may be too painful, and the future too uncertain.

Children of bisexual fathers often feel that Christmas is impossible to deal with. This is usually a conscious family decision, the mother being well aware of her own difficulties as well as those of the children. Anger, sometimes hostility, erupts as the day nears. Irritability is common, and old feelings that remain below the surface for most of the year erupt, causing great pain and distress. Families share similar fears around vacation time. This may be the first time the family would take a vacation without the husband/father, leaving the family upset and abandoned. There is no easy solution to this; learning to live with it becomes less impossible. For some, changing the routine is helpful to lessen the pain.

Disposal of Belongings

A stressful task for the bereaved family is disposing of the deceased person's belongings. Families often have tremendous difficulty searching through and cleaning out personal belongings left behind. These things carry enormously painful but cherished memories. The task can be complicated for families of homosexual men who have to deal with their anger toward the lover, who may have the belongings in his possession, and their feelings of estrangement. This is compounded when the lover and/or the family were not invited to or were prohibited from attending the funeral service.

One wife redecorated her bedroom and turned it into a family room. This minimized charged memories for her, and yet kept the room as an intimate part of the family home.

Visiting the Grave

For most families a visit to the grave is an agonizingly painful ordeal. Some wives experience extreme guilt on preventing the children from visiting the grave, fearing it may trigger a severe reaction with which they are not ready to cope. The avoidance of visiting the grave may be an indication of inhibited grief. Visiting the cemetery, in a case of delayed grief, helps to release feelings that have been locked up.

Although Dan's grief was openly expressed, he requested that the school social worker join him in a visit to his father's grave. This experience allowed Dan to recall some memories of pleasant events he had had with his father.

In the first year after the death, many people find comfort in regular visits to the grave. As Weizman and Kamm (1985) state, it is something you can do physically, with your whole body, and is therefore a valuable form of expression. Visiting the grave of your loved one helps to reinforce the finality of the situation. It is also a symbolic way of having contact with the deceased. This activity stirs up memories and feelings and gives you another chance to express those feelings. In one case, the partner of a man who had died of AIDS told his therapist that the visit to the grave helped him feel comfortable to cry unashamedly and embrace his lover's family of origin. He felt at this moment the comfort of his deceased lover.

ROLE OF SUPPORT GROUPS

Research indicates that social support buffers the impact of stressful life events (Cohen & Willis 1985; Kessler & McLeod 1985; Thoits 1983; Turner 1983). Since effective support often comes from others facing the same stressors (Gottlieb 1978; Thoits 1983), and because of the stigma of AIDS, survivors of persons who died of AIDS may derive particular benefit from involvement in support groups.

Most grieving individuals say that they experience enormous difficulties in finding others in their immediate environment who will allow them the privilege of open expression of emotion and feeling. This has been exacerbated by the stigma of AIDS. Parents and spouses, particularly, often experience a terrible sense that others—even those close to the family—do not really understand the wretched agony they feel in the face of this loss. They seem to sink into the mire of their own grief. They often characterize themselves as "going under" or as being "swept along" in the emotional storm that follows the death, unable to find an anchor. Families reach out to others, only to have those toward whom they reach turn away.

Katz and Bender (1976) define self-help groups as "voluntary, small group structures for mutual aid and the accomplishment of a special purpose":

They are usually formed by peers who have come together for mutual assistance in satisfying a common need, overcoming a common handicap or life-disrupting problem, and bringing about desired social and/or personal change. . . . They often provide material assistance, as well as emotional support; they are frequently cause-oriented, and promulgate an ideology or values through which members may attain an enhanced sense of personal identity. (91)

Some of the significant unacknowledged and unmet emotional and social-psychological needs of family survivors of homosexual and bisexual men can be addressed in such groups. All families we interviewed who had lost a son, husband, sibling or father to AIDS felt that the first time their story was truly heard was by people like themselves who carried the burden of a toxic secret. Particularly important is a support system that challenges, informs and nurtures. Although the families recognized that the group would not fill the void in their lives, the understanding and compassion of group members enabled them to reenter their world with dignity and hope.

Some families feel a strong drive to respond to the death of their loved one in a public way. Often we see strong desires by bereaved parents of homosexual men, less so among wives of bisexuals, to found or to manage organizations. These organizations include those devoted to supporting research on AIDS. These public responses to the death can be understood as an assertion of competence in one's grief and a strong positive contrast to withdrawal.

The social support group becomes a new psychobiologic regulator, and, within that context, families can explore the ways they can meet problems such as how to celebrate the holidays or what to tell others about the cause of death. Just as shared love of the deceased person provides models for the new families, so shared grief provides models for the newly bereaved families.

In their work with bereaved AIDS survivors, clinicians have visited graves with families, lovers and friends, have attended funerals and memorial services. While unorthodox or inappropriate under other circumstances, these activities have proved to be very significant to bereaved persons and have provided them with opportunities and inspiration to confront difficult issues or take forward strides in their treatment.

IMPLICATIONS FOR PRACTITIONERS

There is still much to be learned about the dynamics of intervening with families of homosexual and bisexual men. We have, however, begun to explore some of the complexities of bereavement based on what we know of families. Families are shocked and often devastated by the death of their loved one. Connecting to families where the member died of AIDS requires a good deal of outreach, since for many the stigma has exacerbated their withdrawal from mental health professionals.

Feelings of pain, anger, guilt and helplessness can be relieved considerably during bereavement if prompt and appropriate intervention starts at the time of anticipatory grief and continues through the period of acute grief. The various stages of bereavement and the individual differences in mourning require various treatment techniques.

When counseling family members it is essential for practitioners to learn from each person what meaning they attach to AIDS and to death, and to help them explore alternative interpretations. The process of discovery may redeem the experience, but is likely to be wrenching and painful. Family identity and roles will never be the same following death, and the family must mourn that loss.

Helping families find ways of maintaining a sense of continuity with past history may be especially hard as they experience a painful present and a frightful future. A past history of failed rescue attempts and unresolved guilt may exacerbate present pain. Support from the clinician in working through the impact of failure will go a long way toward alleviating this distress.

It is also possible that with social support and sharing of the grief, the clinician can help families work through their loss. Practitioners can facilitate the family's engagement in self-help and mutual-aid networks. Through these networks, those who believe that people without their experience cannot understand them learn to trust others. Because the timing of the individual family members' bereavement process varies greatly within and between families, it is also important that practitioners meet these survivors where they are and facilitate grief work accordingly. Consideration should be given to the value of networking and of group work with bereaved families.

The self after the resolution of the death of a family member is different than the self was before the death. Such psychic reorganization provides elements for a new self, which can be a rich development in the survivor's life. One cannot work long with bereaved families without realizing the strength and depth of their lives. All ends are also new beginnings.

CHAPTER 7

Intervening with Inner-City Survivors of AIDS

The evolution of AIDS in inner-city communities has followed a completely divergent course from that in the larger or white-majority community. The differences have been physical, social, psychological and economic, and in turn have affected survivors and their experiences of grief and loss. To fully understand the experience of survivorship in African-American and Hispanic communities, it is critical to analyze the impact of AIDS on individuals and families with primary residence in inner-city communities.

Figure 7.1 indicates that African-Americans and Hispanics have suffered a disproportionately large share of the burden of AIDS in the United States. The racial distribution of cases has remained stable over time, with only a few exceptions. For example, AIDS cases in adult white males decreased in 1989 and the reported cases among African-Americans and Hispanics increased.

The ever-expanding number of individuals and families infected with HIV and full-blown AIDS, suggests that the number of survivors is already extensive, and will increase exponentially.

This chapter will address the process of recovery among individuals and families in the inner city from the death of a loved one from AIDS. Clinical interventions will illustrate how professionals can respond in a sensitive manner in working with bereaved inner-city families.

INTRODUCTION

Perhaps the best way to begin this discussion is to define the terms inner-city and ethnicity. Inner-city, in this chapter, refers to those physically deteriorated, urban areas inhabited primarily by indigent African-American

Figure 7.1
Racial Breakdown of Those Who Have Been Diagnosed as Having AIDS in the United States through September 1991

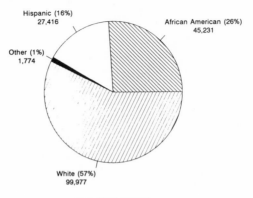

Hispanic (16%)
27,416

Other (1%)
1,774

African American (26%)
45,231

White (57%)
99,977

Male Total 174,398

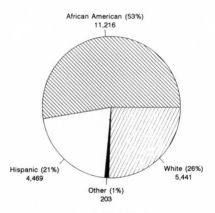

African American (53%)
11,216

Hispanic (21%)
4,469

Other (1%)
203

White (26%)
5,441

Female Total 21,320

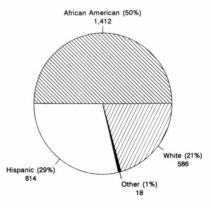

African American (50%)
1,412

Hispanic (29%)
814

Other (1%)
18

White (21%)
586

Pediatric Total 2,830

Source: Centers for Disease Control

and Hispanic populations (Kane 1981; Reissman 1976). A U.S. Department of Health and Human Services task force on black and minority health (1986) describes these regions as:

urban areas characterized by low income, physical deterioration, welfare dependency, racial and ethnic concentrations, broken homes, working mothers, low levels of education and vocational skills, high unemployment, high proportion of single males, overcrowded and substandard housing, low rates of home ownership or single family dwellings, mixed land use, and high population density. (31)

Typically these communities are bereft of services, from supermarkets to mental health clinics, from safe playgrounds to adequate educational institutions.

It takes very little imagination to visualize the havoc these physical conditions constantly wreak on personality development, self-image and sense of personal control, as well as the subjective, more generalized discomfort of residents. As if the persistent reminder of these conditions were not enough, residents of the inner city are bombarded through television, movies, printed media and their own observations as they travel from their communities to work, play or seek needed services. AIDS, with its stigma, physical and psychological devastations and economic demands, poses yet another catastrophe for people of color.

The literature is replete with varying and conflicting definitions of ethnicity and oppressed peoples. Ethnicity is often utilized as a descriptive term. In this context, ethnicity refers to a concept of a group's "peoplehood," uniting those who conceive of themselves as alike by virtue of their common ancestry, real or fictitious, and who are so regarded by others (McGoldrick 1989, 70). It is a personal, self-chosen identity, reflecting a common ancestry, national origin, religion and/or race. Hodges (1989) notes that "ethnicity is reflected by group members assuming similarity in the life styles, values, attitudes, customs and rituals of people in their respective groups" (95).

Minority, a term often used in the older literature, is a descriptive term, employed to define groups that are discriminated against and/or experience differential and unequal treatment because of oppressive conditions (Lum 1986). Although some authors include in their discussions of minority persons all peoples of color, white ethnics (Poles, Greeks, Italians) and/or socioreligious ethnics (Jews, Arabs, Mormons), we reserve this term for African-American and Hispanic people living in the inner city.

There are enormous differences among those included in this definition. Some born in this country, and numerous others migrating from their native countries, retain varying degrees of their original culture and language. Differences exist among African-Americans; some are born and raised in the North, others raised in the rural and urban South and others come to the United States from the West Indies and Africa. Variations within the Hispanic community stem from different origins and commitments to countries in South and Central America and the Caribbean, in addition to those born in this country (LeVine & Padilla 1980). Critical to our discussion is that ethnicity, race and minority status all affect attitudes toward death and the way bereavement is experienced (Dershimer 1990).

THE IMPACT OF AIDS ON INNER-CITY COMMUNITIES

The statistics related to AIDS in inner-city communities present a partial picture (See Figure 7.1). Besides physically depleting the population in such communities, AIDS has been a hard taskmaster, exiling individuals and families from their relatives, friends and significant others. Inner-city families live in physical proximity to neighbors and institutions, where intimate interaction is prevalent and private information or behaviors hard to hide. An individual's diagnosis of AIDS, which promptly and invariably becomes public knowledge, automatically imposes shame and stigma on family relationships and has a negative impact on identity and self-esteem.

The statistics also fail to indicate the numerous and intense stresses that precede and follow the illness and death of a loved one from AIDS. Families and individuals are unable to resolve their grief as they are forced to confront the next crisis or attempt to stave off another approaching disaster. Equally understated is the emotional havoc and devastation that AIDS imposes on families and individuals, already overwhelmed by their efforts to survive and constantly struggling against physical and economic difficulties. The antagonism of bureaucrats and professionals who have considerable involvement with the lives of inner-city residents frequently contributes to, rather than alleviates, problems. Freely used labels such as disadvantaged, impoverished and culturally deprived connote inadequacy rather than appreciation for strengths and for the ability to continue to struggle against intractable societal deficiencies.

According to Walker (1987), each PWA leaves between five and seven survivors—parents, siblings, relatives, lovers, friends and significant others. Since African-Americans and Hispanics tend to have large families, and have adapted various family forms that expand the number of individuals likely to be considered family members (notably extended and augmented families and the emotional recognition of godparents and adoptive children), the number of survivors in this population will be higher.

LOSS, GRIEF AND ETHNICITY

Dershimer (1990) and Stephenson (1985) contend that grief and bereavement are human responses far more powerful and complex than are explicated by contemporary models of grief and loss. The tendency in most of these models (Bowlby 1973, 1980a; Freud 1957; Parkes 1972; Raphael 1983; Worden 1982) is to view grief and bereavement in psychological terms and to recommend psychotherapy as the mode of helping with grief-induced internal stresses.

The relevance of these models must be viewed within the context of an ongoing debate about the usefulness of traditional psychotherapy to poor, inner-city residents in general, and by extension to AIDS survivors in these communities. Some authors believe that long-term psychotherapy is denied inner-city residents because of discrimination, evident in the notion that inner-city clients are incapable of insight therapy and the consequent decision not to waste funds providing such services to them.

In general, the emotional problems of residents in such communities are most commonly treated with short-term models and/or medication rather than with long-term therapy. Rubenstein and Bloch (1982) provide a useful clarification, noting that "reports of practice and some research evidence suggest that even under current discriminatory conditions and without major social change, minority group members need, want and can benefit from interpersonal help that is responsive to their culture, traditions and life experiences" (187).

Thus to be useful, existing models of bereavement must take into consideration social and cultural variables and the unique customs, concerns and responses of African-Americans and Hispanics to loss and grief. This position is supported by a number of authors (Brown 1989; Carter & McGoldrick 1989; Jackson 1980; Kalish & Reynolds 1981; LeVine & Padilla 1980; Stephenson 1985) who assert that culture and ethnicity determine the ways we view death and dying and how we respond to loss and bereavement. Kalish and Reynolds claim unequivocally that "there seems to be little doubt that ethnic background is an important factor in attitudes, feelings, beliefs and expectations that people have regarding dying, death, and bereavement" (49).

Aguilar and Wood (1976), in discussing mourning among persons of Mexican descent, describe the stages of depression, the initiation of mourning (consisting of the wake and the lying in state); acceptance of reality, burial and collective acceptance of reality by family and friends; a second depression, followed by collective condolences; and final acceptance. While this and other paradigms have much in common, Aguilar and Wood differ in the emphases given to selective factors in the grievers' overall responses. For example, they give much less emphasis to the anger and frustration of the survivor than do other theorists, and pay particular attention to the recurring depression and collective support among Mexican-Americans.

Implicit in this perspective is the salience of both psychological and sociological factors in grief reactions, which is corroborated by Bolin's (1982) efforts to develop a model of family recovery from disasters, including bereavement. Bolin notes:

Family recovery must be seen as the outcome of a relatively complex process. Additionally, to conceptualize family recovery, a multivariate model must be developed

Figure 7.2
Conceptual Model of the Psychosocial Impacts of Survivorship

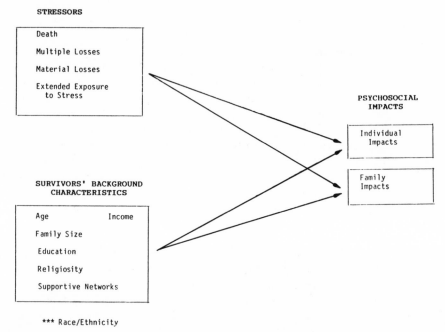

STRESSORS

Death

Multiple Losses

Material Losses

Extended Exposure
to Stress

PSYCHOSOCIAL
IMPACTS

Individual
Impacts

Family
Impacts

SURVIVORS' BACKGROUND
CHARACTERISTICS

Age   Income

Family Size

Education

Religiosity

Supportive Networks

*** Race/Ethnicity

Adapted from Bolin 1982.

since it is unwise to expect a single factor, such as aid, to explain family recovery.
... A good model must give due weight to so-called background characteristics of
the families whose recovery it is trying to explain [and] the variables used must make
sense in light of previous research and be justifiable from a theoretical point of view.
(18)

After reviewing existing models seeking to explain family recovery from
disasters, Bolin presents his own theory and confirms his model through a
systematic study of families recovering from a series of tornadoes.

For our purposes, Figure 7.2 offers a conceptual view of the convergence
of factors critical to the recovery of inner-city residents from the loss of their
loved ones to AIDS. Race and ethnicity, although not fully researched by
Bolin, because "data on minority victims were not available" (31), are essential
factors in a generalized model of recovery.

DYNAMICS OF GRIEF: FAMILIES AND INDIVIDUALS

Leming and Dickinson (1985) note: "While they surely vary, all societies
... seem to have some social mechanism for managing death-related emotions

and reconstructing family interaction patterns modified by death. These customs are passed down from generation to generation and are an integral part of a society's ways of coping with a major event like death" (235).

Our interviews with inner-city survivors of AIDS confirmed the observation that these survivors were, in large measure, remarkably similar to other groups. They were, however, distinguished by the nature and scope of negative socioenvironmental impacts (Lum 1986) to which they were exposed (poverty, racism, specific brand of stigma, cultural taboos, etc.), and by the combined effects of these factors on the bereavement process.

A series of bereavement tasks confronting inner-city survivors emerged in our exploratory interviews with representatives of this population and practitioners who work with them. The tasks, which parallel the needs of the bereaved identified by Sanders (1989), include: dealing with raw emotions, finding meaning in the loss, dealing with practical and legal difficulties, adjusting to a system in transition and finding substitutes for the lost family member.

DEALING WITH RAW EMOTIONS

The loss of a loved one through death is immensely painful. Theorists have consistently identified the feelings associated with death, including sadness, anger, resentment, guilt, fear, shock and anxiety. Simultaneously, thoughts of suicide, withdrawal and helplessness emerge, and the survivor experiences a deep yearning for the pain to cease and for things to revert to the way they were before the death of their loved one. Like all survivors, bereaved inner-city families and individuals experience these emotions when they experience such a loss.

The death of a loved one from AIDS, however, disturbs these families in several unique ways. First it removes a beloved family member at a most inopportune time. Given the nature of the disease, the deceased person is likely to be young, on the verge of becoming productive, independent, financially and emotionally secure. Further, the deceased person may have enormous significance both to the family and the ethnic community. As Carter and McGoldrick (1989) note, "an individual's significance to the family [and to the community] can be understood in terms of the functional role in the family [and the community] and the degree of emotional dependence of the family on the individual" (474).

Second, the stigma associated with AIDS, with persons who die from this disease and their surviving family members hinders, rather than facilitates, the mourning process. Inner-city survivors of persons with AIDS tend to view their deceased loved ones, and, by association, themselves, in triple jeopardy. They all are stigmatized as African-Americans and Hispanics; their deceased loved ones are stigmatized as deviants because of their sexual orientation and/or drug use, and as purveyors of a deadly, sleazy disease (Jue 1987).

Third, the intricate set of social obligations and mourning duties are not accompanied by the usual forms and sources of social support, because of attitudes toward AIDS, sex, homosexuality and drug use in, and external to, inner-city communities. Although grieving is an intensely personal experience, death and loss are also social matters. As Durkheim, quoted in Stephenson (1985, 142) suggested, "mourning is not a natural movement of private feelings wounded by a cruel loss, it is a duty imposed by the group." Typically friends, neighbors and social institutions such as the church and service organizations render support and encouragement to the bereaved. Unfortunately, in the case of a death from AIDS, these sources have been woefully inadequate and are viewed by surviving families as less than satisfactory.

Inner-city families and individuals experience a wide range of emotions typically associated with grief and bereavement. However, there is an absence of consensus in the literature regarding how these emotions are expressed. For example, Kalish and Reynolds (1981) conducted the single most comprehensive study of the attitudes and reactions of four ethnic groups (Anglo-Americans, African-Americans, Japanese-Americans and Mexican-Americans) to the death of a family member. They identified a variety of cultural and ethnic influences on the way loss is perceived and experienced, and reported that "although the ability to express one's grief openly is frequently encouraged by professionals in the mental health field . . . respondents displayed considerable reluctance to do so" (31). Respondents further indicated that while emotional expression was expected and even encouraged in private, public expression was to be constrained and controlled. Carter and Mc-Goldrick (1989), on the other hand, suggest that African-Americans and Hispanics are apt to express emotions associated with grief and bereavement openly, dramatically and immediately.

Our observations clearly indicated that the expressions of grief by inner-city residents are culturally defined and are not familiar to many mental health practitioners, as illustrated in the following case.

A young Hispanic woman left work immediately on being notified that her brother was hospitalized. She arrived at the hospital anxious and concerned, only to be told that her brother died from AIDS within the hour. She immediately started to scream, sob uncontrollably, call out her brother's name over and over again, and finally fell into a seizure-like trance. The medical staff became extremely upset and were uncertain about what to do. A call was made to the social service department, informing the worker that Ms. A. was being transferred to the psychiatric department for further care, and requesting that the worker try to contact and inform other family members. The worker, having some appreciation for cultural dynamics, suggested that she talk to Ms. A. before any actions were taken. The worker remained silent with Ms. A. for sometime, recognizing her severe upset, giving her information about her brother's last hours, and talking quietly until her initial grief abated. Within hours, with the worker's help, Ms. A. had regained her composure, was able to initiate the painful task of informing family members and prepare for an unexpected funeral.

This case reflects the shock and confusion that survivors experience at the moment they become aware of the death of a loved one. It further illustrates the feelings of unreality, the sheer disbelief that the death has occurred, the apprehension and physical symptoms that survivors display. The case of Ms. A. offers a vivid example of the varying cultural expectations that accompany the death of a loved one. Ms. A., having begun the process of mourning, will proceed to experience the range of emotions and to accomplish the various tasks of bereavement, albeit at her own pace and in her unique, culturally defined, way.

The willingness of the worker to assess this case on the basis of Ms. A.'s overt behavior and to utilize an appreciation of cultural factors led to a turning point in this case. The worker allowed, indeed encouraged, Ms. A. to express her shock and anger at the death of her brother in her culturally unique way. The clinician demonstrated an appreciation of Ms. A.'s yearning and searching to comprehend her loss, and of the disorganization and despair Ms. A. undoubtedly felt. With patience, the worker provided information and joined with the client as Ms. A. moved toward acceptance of the death and reorganization.

This case also indicates that many inner-city families need help in having the feelings that emerge with the death of their loved ones from AIDS defined and appreciated within a cultural context. Despite an exhaustive number of how-to books purporting to prepare individuals and families to cope with death, dying and grief, the death of a loved one usually finds people ill-prepared. Inner-city individuals and families, constantly struggling to cope with the general life conditions under which they reside, rarely have the luxury to anticipate the demands of death and grief. Raphael (1984) estimates from his study of widows that a third of all major bereavements result in problems for which professional help is required. Our observations indicated that inner-city residents grieving deaths from AIDS were frequently inhibited in their mourning. The discrepancies between their specific beliefs about levels and forms of mourning and the prevailing norms in society, as well as selected socioenvironmental factors, accounted for many of their inhibitions.

It is imperative that mental health practitioners recognize how mourning duties or prescriptions emerge among inner-city families who are African-American and Hispanic. Chestang (1976), Norton (1978) and Mizio and Delaney (1981), recognizing the pluralistic society in which we function, postulate that African-Americans and Hispanics are part of two systems, which exert major influences on their development, behaviors and self-perception. These systems, to which minority individuals are differentially responsive, are the dominant or larger social unit, referred to as the "sustaining system," and the more immediate family or ethnic community system, identified as the "nurturing system."

The sustaining system is seen as housing the instrumental resources that families and individuals need—the goods and services, the political power, economic resources and related factors that confer status and power. Embedded in the larger, sustaining system is the nurturing system, represented by the close physical and social environments. This system provides a climate for the development of the individual's basic sense of identity, aids in the development, restoration and maintenance of the self-esteem and operates as a buffer against the attitudes and activities of the larger community (Chestang 1976).

Norton (1979) indicates that aspects of the nurturing or the sustaining system assume primacy or fade into the background depending on the experience or situation in which the individual finds himself/herself or the family finds itself. The force and fury of AIDS projects one of these external systems differentially into the forefront. Inner-city individuals and families respond to one system or another depending on various factors. For example, when arranging for funeral services, the survivor may be responsive to the dictates of the larger system. If the survivor does not have the financial resources to pay for an appropriate funeral, the larger social system looms to the forefront in the individual's experience. For the solace and comfort requisite for coping with grief or even to provide the financial resources to underwrite the funeral, the inner-city family may turn to significant and potentially helpful elements in the nurturing system.

The push and pull of the two critical systems is illustrated in the following case:

When Luis died, Mr. and Mrs. Santos, a Hispanic couple, were extremely sad and distraught. At the same time, they were heartened by the fact that they had achieved a reconciliation with their son during the final months of his life. A day after Luis's death, the Santos met with the medical social worker who had known Luis over the course of his hospitalization. They talked about the years they had felt alienated and how guilty they were for not understanding Luis's homosexuality. They stated that they denied his accomplishments. Mr. and Mrs. Santos were convinced that the family ties developed in Luis's early years served to surmount the enormous chasm that developed between them. They were determined to see that his death was not in vain and that the final rites would serve to honor his memory appropriately.

In the worker's presence they opened the envelope Luis had left with his last instructions and learned that he wished to be cremated and have his ashes returned to Puerto Rico. They could not recall anyone in their community who had been cremated and did not even know how to go about making the necessary arrangements. Ms. N., the social worker, listened to their expression of cultural attitudes toward cremation and explored the conflicts between what they would do and what Luis expected. They related their uneasiness about their religious convictions and the reactions they would expect from their friends and neighbors. Ms. N. conveyed her support regarding how difficult it was to follow through on Luis's request, knowing that it was not in keeping with their cultural norms.

She asked how they might respond to questions or comments from friends and neighbors. When they expressed uncertainty, she helped them think and enact what they might say. As they talked further, they were able to state clearly that abiding by Luis's wishes was more important than anything else. They felt encouraged, and that they would be able to follow through with these plans.

When Ms. N. wondered about their talking to someone in the church regarding their religious concerns, Mr. and Mrs. Santos indicated that they were not completely sure what response they might receive. They indicated that in recent months an "espiritista" had been very sympathetic and helpful to them. They agreed that they could visit her to talk about Luis's death and their concerns about the afterlife.

Ms. N.'s appreciation of the influences of the sustaining and nurturing systems was instructive in her assessing how to help Mr. and Mrs. Santos. She did not impose the values of either system, but enabled Mr. and Mrs. Santos to identify which values and positions were currently most important to them. In effect, she empowered Mr. and Mrs. Santos to assume cognitive and behavioral responsibility for their choices, to consider the implications of these choices and how they could implement them, without undue emotional conflict, while they proceeded with the ordinary tasks of bereavement.

FINDING MEANING IN THE LOSS

It is not unusual for survivors to engage in obsessional reviews, in which events surrounding the death of a loved one are relived over and over again in a search for meaning. This quest is more philosophical than pragmatic in that the survivor seeks to make sense of the death (Kastenbaum 1986), not necessarily regarding the cause of death, but regarding its meaning in the overall scheme of things. Since there is no final or practical answer to the question "Why my loved one?" such a question can continue to haunt survivors for indefinite periods of time. In the case of death from AIDS both the question and the quest may linger indefinitely.

In our initial discussion of grief (see Chapter 1), we noted the need for the bereaved person to realize that the loss was important. Losses that are not considered important will not be mourned; losses that are considered important appear to stimulate a more intensive search for the meaning of the death. Similarly, there is general agreement (Parkes & Weiss 1983; Raphael 1984; Osterweis 1984) that the nature of the death can have a debilitating effect on the bereaved person, which in turn complicates the grieving process. In the case of death from AIDS several socioenvironmental factors combine to affect the search for meaning in which inner-city residents engage. Among the principal socioenvironmental factors are the stigma associated with AIDS, poverty, lack of access to health care, racism and the attitude of organized religion toward homosexuality.

Early in the epidemic, few deaths from AIDS were reported or became cause for general concern in African-American and Hispanic communities. Unwittingly, inhabitants in these communities were lulled into thinking that AIDS was the gay, white community's business. Attitudes were further complicated by reports that Africa and Haiti were the locus of origin of the disease. Discrimination against and rejection of persons with AIDS—refusal of medical care, housing, employment benefits and insurance, as well as suggestions that they be quarantined or worse—were regularly reported in the media. Later, surviving relatives and friends witnessed during their loved one's illness the denial of medical and dental care, the refusal of housekeeping personnel to clean hospital rooms, the refusal of admission to schools or educational programs and negative responses from funeral directors. The evidence was clear. PWAs are personae non gratae in the eyes of the general public, health care practitioners and the government responsible for health care and social policies.

It was, and is, within this social context that inner-city survivors of PWAs confront their grief—the sadness and confusion--that they feel, and the mourning or public expression of that grief. Communities and individuals, already stigmatized, now face another, even more socially unacceptable, fatal and complicated onus.

Within this context it is almost impossible for survivors to give any meaning to the death of their loved ones, that is to think of positive features of the deceased person's life or of their mutual relationship and prior experiences. Family members are tempted to deny the very existence or crucial aspects of their deceased loved one or, motivated by anger and resentment, to neglect to follow the deceased person's last wishes. These incidents serve to encourage denial and suppression of the griever's feelings and mourning behaviors.

The following case example gives some understanding of the impact of society on a survivor:

Mrs. P., a fifty-eight-year-old African-American woman, had been attending a group of mothers of PWAs for several weeks. She found this experience extremely gratifying and helpful in understanding the dilemmas associated with being a caregiver of a PWA, in reestablishing communication with her gay son from whom she had been alienated, and in preparing for his eventual death. Despite extensive intellectual preparation, when he died, Mrs. P. was emotionally devastated and found her group members particularly helpful with planning and implementing the details of her son's funeral and carrying out his wishes for an open coffin during the service.

At the meeting immediately following his death and before his burial, she reported on a discussion with the funeral director. She strongly felt that in her African-American community, the expectation was that there be an open coffin during the funeral, but found herself torn and upset about what to do. She had been unable to call relatives who should be coming for the funeral. She could not understand why the funeral director was so aggressive in trying to convince her that she should plan for a closed coffin. While encouraging Mrs. P. to insist on her preference and to feel comfortable with her view, the group members explained that, out of irrational fears of being infected, the funeral director was unwilling to prepare the body for an open viewing. The group helped her to appreciate the stigma and discrimination operative in his behavior.

This group, active, verbal and fully immersed in the mutual aid process, is different from some other groups for inner-city survivors, which place less emphasis on verbalizing feelings, open communication and direct confrontation (Jue 1987). In order for groups of this kind to be helpful, practitioners must aid and abet group members early in the process, model the helping process and encourage individuals to share their concerns.

The worker here accepted the descriptions of situations and reached for Mrs. P.'s readiness to link her feelings and thoughts with the words. The worker enabled the group to be mindful of the importance for Mrs. P. of expressing her grief in culturally desirable ways and of gaining a perspective on the motivations of the funeral director. Mrs. P.'s activities and decisions at this time were enormously important in determining how she would proceed with grieving and mourning her son—with finding the capacity to give meaning to his life and to her relationship with him.

The importance of the deceased family member and the meaning given to his or her death are likely to be felt differently by different members. Practitioners may become aware that family members, so occupied with their own grief, may be unable to console other family members or meet the needs of children and adolescents. Grief is an individual process, which means that the pace for each member will be individually defined, and, more than likely, out of sync with the pace of other family members.

When the deceased family member is considered important by one or some family members and not by others, the imbalance is likely to create disagreement and conflicts within the family. These dissatisfactions may complicate the grieving process for all mourners, as illustrated in the following case.

Mrs. Y., an African-American woman and a long-term user of illicit substances, abandoned her three children, leaving them with her boyfriend, who had lived with them for a decade. Mr. P. loved the children, and with the help of a social worker and financial assistance from the Child Welfare Administration (CWA), had managed to make a home for them. In the two years that she was away, Mrs. Y. made several calls, usually when she was high on one or another substance and two visits, which had been enormously tense and unsatisfactory to all involved.

When she became ill with AIDS and was hospitalized, she requested that the medical social worker call the CWA social worker. During the initial visit, Mrs. Y. wanted the worker to know about her illness so that they could arrange for the children to be cared for permanently by Mr. P. rather than by members of her biological family or in foster care. The CWA worker acknowledged Mrs. Y.'s illness and the difficulties she was facing and inquired about how she was managing and the care she was receiving. The worker also supported Mrs. Y.'s concern for her children at this critical time in her life and noted how important this concern would be to the children. Mrs. Y. and the worker talked extensively about the legal and social arrangements that would be required. They agreed that the current home situation was good for the children and that the worker would follow up by talking with Mr. P. and the family.

During the second visit, Mrs. Y. asked about the children and sought details on how they were managing. The worker answered her questions, and was not surprised when Mrs. Y. requested to see the children during the next visit. The worker recognized Mrs. Y.'s yearning and her wish to see them before she died. She explored how Mrs. Y. thought the visit would go. Though she could not promise that the children would visit the next time, she agreed to discuss the plans with Mr. P. and the children. Together, Mrs. Y. and the worker, with some input from Mr. P., would assess the children's readiness to make the hospital visit. The worker explored what Mrs. Y. wanted to share with the children about her illness and her future plans and together they considered how Mrs. Y. might respond to some of the difficult questions the children might ask.

The worker arranged to make a visit to Mr. P.'s home. When she broached the subject with Mr. P. he was immediately adamant against any in-person contacts. He railed with anger against Mrs. Y's behavior in abandoning the children: "She now wants to use them to satisfy her whims." The worker allowed Mr. P. to vent his anger, and asked about his own thoughts about the children's future. The worker explored his feelings about having these decisions thrust on him as well as his anger over Mrs. Y.'s abandonment. The worker then wondered aloud whether the children should be a part of the decision. Mr. P. and the worker agreed that they would jointly tell the children and consider whether a visit to Mrs. Y. would be in their best interests.

Mr. P. invited Jeremy, seventeen years old, Beth, ten years old and Ann, twelve years old, to talk with him and the worker. In the meeting, Jeremy expressed his anger and was completely against going to see his mother. He reiterated his step-father's sentiment, that his mother had abandoned them. "She left us then, now it is our time to refuse to see her. She had it coming, and I don't feel any sympathy for her." Initially, Beth and Ann were silent, and it was obvious that they were unsure about how to respond. Beth asked, "How sick is my mother? How is she managing? Does she really want to see us?"

The worker validated Beth's concern about her mother and talked about how sick Mrs. Y. was. Ann said, "Part of me wants to see my mother and a part of me does not. Since Jack (Mr. P.) told us about your visit, Beth and I have been talking about my mother." The worker normalized their ambivalence and allayed their fears about the visit. She spent the remaining time exploring their worries and concerns and stated that the decision to visit was really up to them. The worker suggested a follow up session which would give them time to think about the issues and feelings that were raised. They called within a week to say that they had thought about it and would like to use the next visit to see Mrs. Y.

The worker picked up the family, including Mr. P., and used the travel time to prepare them for the visit and to allay their remaining fears and anxieties. Although the visit was tense, it was a beginning for Mrs. Y. and the family to talk about the losses they had and would experience.

Mrs. Y. died a week later. It was the worker who went to the home to tell the family. She spent the time talking about Mrs. Y.'s death. Follow-up visits with the children and Mr. P. focussed on their grieving and on permanency planning.

The worker's role in this case, beginning with efforts to help Mrs. Y. achieve her last requests, was to act as a catalyst in helping the family prepare for death and mourn the enormous losses they had experienced repeatedly throughout the children's lives. The socioenvironmental impacts, primarily their poverty, were evident in this case, and although not fully described, there can be no question but that this family had been exposed to stresses and demands above and beyond their capacities. They were fortunate to have the assistance of an understanding and competent social worker in confronting their concrete needs—for money, housing, health care and so on—but this situation may well have been an exception.

This case is a good example of Carter and McGoldrick's (1989) observation that "an individual's significance to the family can be understood in terms of the functional role in the family and the degree of emotional dependence of the family on the individual" (147). Despite Mrs. Y.'s lack of involvement with her children and her failures in parenting them, an emotional connection still existed between them, one that facilitated their anticipatory mourning, but had to be resolved in some way before and after her death.

Aguilar and Wood (1976) identify the burial and collective condolences as one of the particular stages in the bereavement process for Hispanics. The significance of funerals for African-Americans and Hispanics, who generally consider death the most significant life cycle transition (Carter & McGoldrick 1989), is reflected in their attitudes toward and behaviors related to these rituals. Carter and McGoldrick (1989) observe that "family members are expected to make every effort to attend a relative's or friend's wake and funeral. Black families in the South often incur great expenses to have flowers, a band, singing and other accompaniments for the funeral. Funerals are delayed for days to make sure that all family members can get there" (81).

Claude Brown, in his autobiographical novel, *Manchild in the Promised Land* (1965), paints the picture of mourning expectations more colorfully, but no less informatively:

The best [church] songs were sung at the funerals for "bad niggers." I learned that a bad nigger was a nigger who didn't take shit from nobody and that even the "crackers" didn't mess with him.

One day I went to a funeral for a bad nigger. A lot of people were there, and most of them had heard about him but were seeing him for the first time. I guess they were scared to see him while he was still alive and still bad. . . . At his funeral, a lot of ladies cried and the preacher talked about him real loud for a long time. Before the preacher started talking, somebody sang "Before This Time Another Year" and

"Got on My Traveling Shoes." When the preacher finished talking about him, they took the casket outside and put it down in the ground. I had seen people do that before, but I didn't think they would do it this time. It just didn't seem like the right way to treat a bad nigger, unless being dead made him not so bad any more. . . . Somebody would sing real good at Grandpa's funeral, and a lot of people would be there. It would have to be a big funeral, because Grandpa was a real bad evil nigger when he was a young man. (48–49)

Kalish and Reynolds (1981) offer a glimpse of mourning behaviors associated with the Hispanic community in their description of "the funeral of a Mexican American who was well known and highly esteemed in the San Diego area for his work in helping farm workers' children attend college":

He was killed in an automobile accident. At the churchyard, the mourners who had followed the procession from the church remained after the priest said prayers at the graveside and left. The cemetery caretaker, not himself Mexican American, forbade them from staying while the coffin was lowered into the ground, a rule at the cemetery. A few left, but the majority remained. A mourner brought out his guitar and began to play a piece that the dead man had particularly liked; others also played the guitar and sang, with the mourners at times joining in as a group, many of them through streams of tears. Finally the Anglo caretaker returned and said "You people have to leave—if you don't I'll call the police." The mourners became angry and refused to leave until they felt ready. (178)

Funerals serve a range of different purposes. They serve to confirm and reinforce the reality of loss for the survivors. Simultaneously, they assist in giving meaning to the loss as they provide an expression of the community's respect for and appreciation of the deceased. Family members, cognizant of the stigma and attitudes toward AIDS, may be uncertain about whether to plan a private or more public event to honor their deceased member. The nature of the reactions of others, communication of sympathy and condolences, the participation in the funeral all promote community support for the survivors and acknowledge the importance of the person who has died.

DEALING WITH PRACTICAL AND LEGAL DIFFICULTIES

The realities of life and the demands of daily living continue during the process of grief and mourning. Throughout this process there may be a range of practical problems concerning finances, housing, caring for children, handling funeral arrangements and legal problems related to planning for permanent child care or the disposal of property. The clinician may have to take an active and direct role as liaison with other agencies and in sorting out the practical difficulties. It may become necessary for the clinician to help the bereaved person take direct action (for example in deciding on funeral arrangements) by providing advice or relevant information. For instance, the worker might have assisted Mr. P. in the case mentioned earlier with adopting the children in keeping with Mrs. Y.'s last wishes.

Economic and employment problems often plague inner-city AIDS survivors, complicating an already painful existence characterized by constant confrontation with poverty, racism and discrimination. Some of our respondents reported having to take vacation time to attend to their ill family member or to attend the funeral of their loved ones, or having to return to work before they felt ready. In general they had to maintain a cloak of secrecy in their work environment regarding the cause of death. Stephenson (1985) describes this situation well:

When one must return to work before the [grieving] process is complete, a great deal of effort must be expended by the individual to maintain a facade of nonemotionality. It may be necessary for the person to deny his or her feelings in order to continue to function in the world of work. Something of one's humanness must be sacrificed in order to bring home the paycheck. This imposition of behaviors on the mourner may be a product of the bureaucratic form of organization. In the bureaucracy, death is not known. (146)

African-American and Hispanic survivors of PWAs operate in stark fear of losing their jobs or facing greater economic stresses as well as of being devoid of the typical support and sympathy generally extended to mourners. With limited resources (such as savings) or transferable skills, the loss of a job has greater significance for individuals and families in this population.

Sometimes the inner-city bereaved may face the problem of what to tell children about the death of a parent from AIDS. This is an area in which many relatives and friends may be keen to give conflicting advice, failing to appreciate the stigma and unconventional nature of this death. Bereaved persons should be helped to think about the implications of any course of action, including planning what they will say and anticipating any repercussions, and responses to these repercussions.

Work with inner-city families and individuals may include the provision of information, advice and tangible supports (for example, underwriting the transportation of an important family member); the expression of feelings, acting as a communication link where individuals are in danger of becoming isolated; and guiding the clarification of problems and the consideration of solutions. The following case example reflects the need for skillful clinical and environmental interventions.

Sam, a fourteen-year-old African-American adolescent, was away at camp for the first time in his life when his father died suddenly from AIDS. Sam was told of the death by the camp counselor, and, although saddened, was advised to continue his stay at camp. Sam was very conflicted, because he had seen funerals previously in his Harlem community. He knew that relatives who had not visited for years came from all parts of the country, and neighbors brought food and were very attentive to the children. He also had a sense that others would be wondering where he was, and that he would be seen as having fun when others were mourning. He wished that he could have talked with someone about these feelings, but didn't have the confidence to raise the subject with his friends or the counselor.

By the time he returned, the funeral service had been held, and the rest of the family were handling their grief relatively isolated from each other. He came back to an environment in which no one was willing to talk about what had happened or to tell him any details about the death and funeral. The family was surprised and disappointed when Sam became progressively more angry, withdrawn from others, and expressed negative feelings about his father.

Finally, when the family was forced to take him to see a social worker at the local mental health clinic, Sam told the worker that he felt as if he had imagined the whole thing. The worker recognized that he had not been able to find a way of expressing his grief or gaining comfort from other members of the family. The worker's first task was to help the family gain some sense of how Sam viewed the situation and how they were coping with their own grief. This was not easily accomplished since this inner-city family felt that one simply dealt with death and that talking about it only made one feel sadder and didn't bring the deceased back.

The worker recognized the crisis nature of Sam's situation and convinced the family that he should see Sam for a series of individual sessions. In these meetings he enabled Sam to ask questions about death, his father's illness and death, and why his family was behaving the way it did. The worker helped Sam normalize his fears, allowed him to cry and to express his anger and sadness and his fears about being infected.

As Sam's behavior in school and at home improved, the family became more amenable to talking with the worker. He successfully engaged them in sessions where they were able to talk about their feelings and to share them with Sam. They brought out some pictures that friends had taken at the funeral and agreed to take Sam to his father's grave, both of which enabled him to grasp the reality of what had happened and gave some meaning to his father's death, at a level that was appropriate for Sam's stage of development and personality.

According to Norton (1978), the sustaining system (represented by the immediate community, friends and neighbors) was supposed to act as a buffer against the attitudes and activities of the larger system and to restore and maintain the self-esteem of its members. Unfortunately for inner-city families, in the case of AIDS much of the stigma characteristic of the larger social system is replicated in the immediate ethnic communities. Dalton (1989) and Jue (1987) have reported the long-standing homophobia and ambivalence toward drug use in both African-American and Hispanic communities. In both situations the behaviors and life-styles have been clearly condemned, while individual gays and drug users may be fully accepted as long as their "deviant" behavior is not flaunted and the communities are not pushed to the wall for broader acceptance.

Within the African-American and Hispanic communities, individuals who are gay are expected to downplay, if not hide, their sexual orientations. The notion of gay pride is nonexistent, requiring minority gays to join the white gay community for acceptance or to remain isolated. Homosexuality is viewed as perverted and obscene, a disease to be cured or a sin against God and nature. Positive role models are notoriously absent, and many gay African-American and Hispanic men are forced to adopt a macho stance, assume the appearance of straight men and to become (or appear to be) intimately and sexually involved with women.

With respect to drug use, the dilemmas are clearly suggested in Dalton's (1989) observations:

> We as a community have a complex relationship with illicit drugs, a relationship that often paralyzes us. On the one hand, blacks are scared to even admit the dimensions of the problem for fear that we will all be treated as junkies and our culture viewed as pathological. On the other, we desperately want to find solutions. For us, drug abuse is a curse far worse than you can imagine. Addicts prey on our neighborhoods, sell drugs to our children, steal our possessions and rob us of hope. We despise them. We despise them because they hurt us and because they are us. They are a constant reminder of how close we all are to the edge. And "they" are "us" literally as well as figuratively; they are our sons and daughters, our sisters and brothers. (217)

This viewpoint and its implications also apply to the Hispanic community. These communities were devoid initially of information concerning AIDS (forms of transmission, experimental drugs, preventive data and techniques, etc.). The health care organizations set up to educate and assist PWAs and survivors mostly serve white gay communities (for example, Gay Men's Health Crisis, buddy programs, etc.). Perhaps the most unfortunate factor is that bisexual practices in minority communities are encouraged by homophobia and the emphasis on machismo. As a result, women who become partners of bisexuals and drug users are inadvertently and unknowingly exposed to the AIDS virus. Now these women and their children are becoming the new group of PWAs, facing death and leaving their own cadre of survivors.

There is extensive theoretical support for the idea that the bereavement process is facilitated when individuals and families have and can turn to friends and other community resources for assistance, emotional support and empathy (Lopata 1979; Raphael 1983; Vachon et al. 1980). Bereavement and loss from AIDS characteristically produce isolation, self-blame and disengagement. In large measure, the behaviors of friends indicate a cultural paranoia, revealed by the subtle expression of negative attitudes and sentiments by potentially supportive figures. Families and individuals from the inner city, already stigmatized and having suffered the brunt of racism and discrimination, may be fearful of exposing themselves to assume still another stigma by admitting the cause of death of their loved ones.

Clinicians may need to advocate, and in selective situations, develop the necessary community resources, and assist the bereaved in identifying existing social supports. In assisting inner-city family members, clinicians should be mindful of Dershimer's (1990) warning that social support should not be interpreted to mean just attention to emotional needs. Dershimer identifies some areas of support that have particular import for inner-city families bereaved from AIDS:

- Helpful information and knowledge (financial management, in addition to baby-sitting and household management)
- Helpful information and knowledge about the general impact of grief (what is considered to be typical grieving, "how to" information for better personal and family functioning)
- Opportunities to reflect on and benefit from religious and spiritual beliefs
- Reaffirmation of significant and comforting values and beliefs
- Reflection on and affirmation of shared norms that provide meaning
- Empowerment of abilities so as to become more self-reliant at critical times
- Encouragement to express emotions (28).

Role of the Church

The role of the church in ethnic communities merits serious consideration. Historically the Protestant churches in African-American communities and the Catholic church in Hispanic communities have occupied unique positions and assume a critical role in serving these populations. The African-American church has been a stabilizing force in family and community life since slavery, and continues to be a significant influence in the lives of inner-city residents (Boyd-Franklin 1989). The church has been, and continues to be, the context in which many secular institutions developed. It is the original African-Americans self-help institution and a safe place for emotional release. The church provides spiritual leadership and emotional and financial supports. Participants are offered opportunities for educational advancement, socialization and participation in social change activities. This institution represents, for active participants, a viable extended family. Indeed, in most inner-city African-American churches, participants refer to each other as Brother and Sister, reflecting an overt commitment to family-like relationships.

Hispanics frequently blend traditions from the Roman Catholic church with practices from their African and Indian heritage into contemporary expressions of faith and spiritual values. These blended values influence the commitment and utilization of religious rituals for birth, marriage and death, and the use of curanderos, spiritists and traditional folk healers in coping with life's crises and problems.

Attitudes among religious individuals toward homosexuality and drug use vary widely. The debates within denominations about homosexuality suggest that selected individuals are demanding changes. The churches as a whole, however, with their marked disapproval of homosexuality, are not very supportive and useful to families and individuals who have survived their loved ones' death from AIDS.

This current withdrawal of the church in both African-American and Hispanic communities is particularly crucial, since it has historically constituted a major social support, primarily in times of grief and bereavement. The criticism has been lodged that "the black [or Hispanic] church has stood in the way of effective AIDS education because of its opposition on moral grounds to homosexuality and drug use" (Dalton 1989, 210). This criticism is only partly valid. It is true that ethnic churches tend to be doctrinally fundamentalist and socially conservative. However, in many communities the concern of an individual church may supercede the theological and philosophical traditions. A family known to the pastor and members of a particular church may receive the sympathy and empathy not publicly expressed or awarded to another more distant community member. The needs of an individual or family member may be so poignantly expressed that representatives of the church might be persuaded to put aside their prejudices for the moment. The major point is that clinicians cannot make a priori judgments about the availability of support from the church to a particular bereaved person without clarifying this reality or assessing whether the griever perceives that support to be available and useful.

ADJUSTING TO A SYSTEM IN TRANSITION

Once the raw emotions of grief have lessened and the bereaved person has begun to accept the reality of the loss, the effort of adjustment becomes a priority. Most individuals find interest in restoring some order to their lives. However, previous patterns of interaction, activities shared with the deceased person and taken-for-granted aspects of life no longer exist, or cease to have meaning. A drastic change in daily routines must be established. The bereaved person is usually ambivalent about completely letting go of the deceased person and needs to separate to establish a new identity without the loved one. Consequently, the point of recognition of the finality of death may be the most difficult period for the bereaved person.

As with other phases of reorganization, socioenvironmental impacts seriously affect both the readiness and capacity of inner-city families to make the requisite adjustment. Theoreticians have developed the concept of "bereavement overload," referring to the overwhelming sense of loss stimulated by multiple deaths. Inner-city families and individuals, particularly because of the disorganization inherent in poverty, are likely to find themselves experiencing fewer stable social supports than those experienced by residents in other communities. They may suffer similar forms of overload caused by losses in employment or housing; decreased emotional ties to friends and neighbors, or friends leaving the neighborhood; or changes with schools such as being transferred to a new school, or the loss of a curriculum with which the child and family were beginning to feel comfortable. Other losses are occasioned by the incessant violence and homicide that characterize life in poor communities.

The intersection of past losses with current ones, the constant and wide-ranging demands of daily life for oppressed people, and the extreme stress occasioned by the death of a loved one from AIDS are sufficient to tax the resources of any family, limiting its ability to adjust. It is critical that the practitioner explore the number and impact of previous losses by making a particular effort to assess the degree of resolution of these losses, both actual and symbolic.

Our interviews with inner-city residents appear to confirm the findings of Sanders (1980) that how bereaved people coped with the stress of previous losses is related to their capacity to adjust to life without the deceased person. The bereaved make adjustments that are very individual. Some families attempt to keep daily routines, physical arrangements and important customs as similar as possible to those of the past. Other families distribute tasks among the remaining family members. Still others attempt to develop com-pletely new routines and to make things as different as possible from the past.

As with other bereavement tasks, resources, information and previous successes—often notoriously unavailable to inner-city residents—facilitate the adjustment. Irrespective of the approach taken by the bereaved persons to adjust, it is evident that time for continued healing and the presence of social supports are important factors in their efforts during the transition period. It is also evident that those families that can be viewed as adjusting create a new system, which will eventually be different from their original family pattern.

Our opportunity to interview inner-city males was quite limited. However, practitioners who work with these families indicated that males appear to have more difficulty making the adjustment to the deaths of their wives and children than do female partners. Clinicians support the view that inner-city men tend to feel a greater need for a sense of control over reality, which precludes their seeking or readily using opportunities to share the events of the death of their loved ones or to talk about personal reactions. Men tend to cut off obsessional reviews through which they could find or attribute meaning to the death, are not as tolerant of dwelling on the past as women are and are less likely to speak openly of their feelings than are women. Perhaps, convinced about the need to provide for basic needs or fearful of losing their jobs, inner-city men may push themselves to return to work earlier than they might ordinarily, and to workplaces that are not naturally supportive or understanding of the need for emotional expression.

These observations should alert clinicians to the need to reach out to males who experience the death of a loved one to AIDS, and to be mindful of the cultural and ethnic issues that affect their adjustment or their efforts to adjust to a system in transition.

FINDING SUBSTITUTES

Families expect, and are expected by society, to meet the physical and emotional needs of their members. The loss of one member leaves a gap in the means and process of fulfilling the needs of surviving family members, until there is a replacement or substitute. Inner-city families, extended as they tend to be, have access to a range of substitutes. However, the probability is that those extended members have previously been assigned supportive roles and functions, and can become overtaxed in times of crises. AIDS, and death from this disease, creates unique crises, the responses to which may be hindered by attitudes of these extended family members. Their antipathy to homosexuality and drug usage, their religiosity, which may preclude full acceptance of the behaviors associated with AIDS and even their irrational fears of contracting the disease may seriously hinder their potential and capacity for enhancing family members' bereavement and adjustment.

A study by Glick, Weiss and Parkes (1974) indicates that, after death, a new cast of helpers appears to replace prior supportive community sources. The needs of the bereaved persons appear to influence the development of helping networks. Some friends and relatives are more instrumental in offering support during the acute or early phase of bereavement, while others are better able to stick with the family for the long run. Raphael (1983) indicates that it is not simply the availability of friends and family members that is important, but how helpful the griever perceives them to be.

Practices and customs in ethnic and religious communities tend to facilitate the development of substitutes to provide for family and individual needs. As bereaved persons begin to gain self-confidence, self-esteem and a perspective on the death of their loved ones, they are able to appreciate and benefit from the efforts of substitutes—persons who can offer some of the emotional support and concrete assistance formerly offered by the deceased person. Practitioners can facilitate the identification and utilization of substitutes by helping bereaved persons sort out who they can trust, what needs they can meet on their own and how they can continue to function with other forms of connectedness.

For African-American and Hispanic families, the deceased loved ones are the sons and daughters who are extensions of the parent, on the one hand, and the hope for the family's and the ethnic community's future, on the other. They are often individuals who have exceeded the achievements of other family members, possessing intellectual or career promise and embodying many of the family's hopes and expectations. The disappointment of not having this promise fully realized and the premature dashing of the family's dreams and hopes make it difficult to accept substitutes.

It is important that practitioners, cognizant of these theoretical constructs and their utility, be flexible in their approach to inner-city ethnic minority families. Bereaved persons may need time before they are ready to accept substitutes. Clinicians should be aware that the definition of a family may be broader than the nuclear family, or family of procreation. Similarly, the substitute for the deceased person may come from a variety of sources and individuals—some with no physical tie to the family—and in various ways.

IMPLICATIONS FOR PRACTITIONERS

Mental health intervention with AIDS survivors in general has been insufficient and even more so with inner-city survivors. Several factors account for this gap in service provision. Utilization of mental health services by poor African-Americans and Hispanics has consistently reflected a mixed picture. They are underrepresented in mental health facilities, less likely than other groups to receive intensive or extensive psychotherapy, more likely to drop out of treatment and more likely to be seen in large, public facilities (Miller 1983).

Mental health practitioners are unlikely to encounter inner-city survivors of PWAs in traditional clinics seeking help with the symptoms of pathological or complicated grief. If anything, such clients are likely to be seen in the social service departments of general hospitals (often with medical problems related to their grieving), agencies serving families and children or public welfare departments. These clients are confronted with such crises as the inability to pay for the funeral of a child deceased from AIDS; insufficient funds to pay for Grandma Duncan's trip from Memphis to attend the funeral of her only grandchild; inordinate and inappropriate demands from a discriminatory funeral director, who may be expressing his prejudice against someone deceased from AIDS, or worse, may be trying to take advantage of the grieving family; facing a job jeopardy hearing because of time taken off to attend to the deceased person during his illness.

Irrespective of the setting in which inner-city AIDS survivors are seen, or the reason that brings them to the attention of the mental health practitioner, to understand fully the responses of inner-city families or individuals to the loss of a loved to AIDS, the clinician must appreciate the dynamic interplay of psychological, social, cultural, economic, political and religious factors and their implications for coping with grief. In effect, the mental health practitioner must assume an ecological perspective to assessment and intervention.

In an epidemic such as AIDS, selective issues—for example, the availability of health care services, the stance of political and religious leaders to AIDS and services to those affected--become crucially important for inner-city individuals and families, or may assume primacy at various times during the grieving process. Priority issues often include: helpful information about the disease, and about the vulnerability of other family members to transmission; the extent and expressions of stigma currently operative, both in the ethnic community and the larger society; and how to avoid self-blame, which often is counterproductive. These items should be covered early in the process.

Glick, Weiss and Parkes (1974) note that a supportive network that may be optimally helpful at one point in time may be dysfunctional at another time. When the opportunity presents itself, it may thus be necessary for a mental health practitioner to make a critical differential assessment of the availability and usefulness of elements in the support system. Clinicians will have to ascertain whether she or he may have to intervene directly in the larger social system. In making treatment decisions, the practitioner will have to be mindful that the grievers' perception of how helpful or available friends and family members are may influence their readiness to utilize professional intervention.

Survivors in general need to feel that their deceased loved ones are accepted as worthwhile individuals, that the loved ones' deaths are recognized as acceptable and that their grief is socially sanctioned. Without these assurances, it becomes exceedingly difficult for individuals to achieve a healthy adjustment to the death and to complete their grief work, returning with self-confidence to society. Given the stigma against AIDS that persists, ethnic minority survivors of PWAs are deprived of these assurances. Rather, with a family member dead from AIDS, many are forced to resort to hiding the true nature of the cause of death, and thus participate in a conspiracy of silence.

Inner-city individuals and families have a pattern of interaction with mental health professionals that is informed by cultural variables and experience. Culturally, these individuals are trained to seek assistance from family members, friends, their regular physicians or church-related helpers, be they ministers, priests, folk healers, spiritists or herbalists. Community ideology involves the notion that mental health services are reserved for the severely mentally ill. The experiences of inner-city residents with utilization of these services have not always been pleasant or productive; stories abound within these communities about the preferential treatment given to others, the insults that ethnic minority individuals have had to endure or the extended period required for any resolution of the problem.

As if the above obstacles to mental health services were not sufficient, in the epidemic of AIDS, the fear and the toxic stigma, the sense of being blamed as a group for the origin and spread of the disease, the absence of the resources and the pride typically found in the gay white community, the slow pace at which the public health establishment has intervened and attempted to identify helpful medications and a cure for the disease, as well as the perspective circulating within these communities that AIDS may be a deliberate act of genocide perpetrated against them, all conspire to make inner-city individuals and families reluctant to seek help.

To counteract these obstacles, clinicians, administrators and policymakers will need to consider ethnic and cultural variables in efforts to attract and hold on to ethnic minority clients who need and can use their services. Systematic and culturally sensitive efforts to reach out to these families must be an essential part of a comprehensive mental health program.

CHAPTER 8

Intervening with Gay Lovers and Friends

Over the course of the AIDS epidemic many gay men have reexamined their behaviors and reconfigured their relationships with lovers and friends. To meet their needs for support, comfort, affection and shared grief, many gay men have decided to engage in monogamous relationships and find strength in one another to buffer the stresses of illness and multiple deaths. At the same time, they have had to adapt and change behaviors and sexual attitudes. Gay men have had lovers, close friends and acquaintances die from AIDS. Concomitantly, they daily confront terminal illness and death, resulting in increased isolation from expected sources of support.

The epidemic has pushed death and mourning to the forefront; many gay men anticipate their own death, and mourn the loss of those close to them. Depending upon their stage of coming out and length of time living a gay life-style, some have had to mourn the loss of old ways of forming emotional and sexual attachments with other men. Because of the social taboos against homosexuality, AIDS and death, gay men are triply stigmatized.

In the last decade an extensive literature has evolved about grief, but until very recently, little or no recognition has been given to the grief of homosexual men who survive the death of a partner or a friend. Recent theoretical and clinical attention to AIDS and the special problems of homosexual partners of persons with AIDS has resulted in renewed interest in the needs of survivors in relationships that continue to lack social approval. Although rampant homophobia continues to be a major social issue, there has been a simultaneous increase in tolerance and recognition of the needs of gay persons whose partners and friends have died from the disease.

Loss, in such large numbers, for gay mourners is new. The increasing number of deaths caused by AIDS among gay men has resulted in an in-

creasing number of survivors who confront the effects of grief and bereavement. Although other segments of the population are affected, gay men are
currently the largest group and have experienced the highest death rate
(Centers for Disease Control 1990a). Due to the numerous losses in some
gay male social networks, emotional expressions associated with grief cannot
be fully experienced before another close friend or lover dies. The specialized
needs of gay men who survive the death of a lover or close friend to AIDS
will be the focus of this chapter.

After discussing grief and bereavement precipitated by the loss of a partner
or friend, we will elaborate on the major stressors, both emotional and practical, that gay survivors experience. Whether the couple lived in a long-term
secret relationship or one of open, public acknowledgment, the death of a
partner represents the ending of a major source of satisfaction. During our
interviews with bereaved gay lovers and friends, the following six issues
emerged: (l) recovering after the death; (2) guilt and other psychological
reactions; (3) personal vulnerability; (4) role of family and friends; (5) social
supports and (6) "moving on."

These bereavement themes have had an impact on the resolution of grief
in nontraditional, gay relationships. We will consider some common manifestations of complicated bereavement and offer suggestions for intervening
with bereaved gay men. We will describe treatment issues related to family,
secret survivorship, self-care and life-style changes using case examples to
elucidate the impact of death from AIDS.

It would be misleading to discuss these six themes without acknowledging
the gay movement and its impact on homosexuals and their behaviors and
attitudes. Large numbers of gay men and women have forged a positive
identity and a sense of self as a source of strength in confronting stigma,
discrimination, rejection by family and society and the overwhelming effects
of AIDS. Drawing on support and sustenance in the gay community, many
have transcended the loss of long-term companions and multiple friends with
dignity.

Practitioners must keep in mind that gay men have frequently chosen not
to disclose their sexual orientation and are not connected to the gay community because of the traditional view of homosexuality as a pathological,
psychological condition. For numerous reasons they are isolated from friends
and relatives, and confront their losses and grief alone. It is this group whom
Siegal and Hoefer (1981) has in mind when they note that the homosexual
person's only support is often the mental health professional. Appreciating
this professional responsibility, our aim is to enhance awareness of the need
for specialized support among this population, and to promote the development of effective interventions.

OVERVIEW

Despite difficulties in determining the true incidence in the general population, it is currently estimated that approximately 10% of the U.S. pop-

ulation is homosexual (Bell & Weinberg 1978). To date, approximately 56,000 deaths have occurred among male homosexuals (Centers for Disease Control 1990a). In spite of these numbers, homosexual concerns have generally been overlooked in the bereavement literature. Fudin and Devore (1981) note that "generally the nuclear family is the conceptual framework within which bereavement is viewed" (132). Theorists considering the counseling needs of survivors have focussed on the loss of a spouse, a child or a parent in the traditional family (Jackson 1979; Miller 1985; Thorson 1985, Dane 1989, 1990).

The survivor in a long-term homosexual relationship does not fall neatly into the primary or secondary categories of survivors established by Keith (1981). Primary survivors consist of spouse, children, siblings and parents. Secondary survivors are close friends. The relationship of primary and secondary survivors to the deceased person are publicly acknowledged. These survivors are granted license to grieve openly in society. Kinship seems to be the principal criterion for legitimacy of grief and mourning. In the case of gay survivors, where few guidelines have been established and few places are available for support and understanding, there is no legitimacy and no public acknowledgment of the grievers.

Homosexuality can be traced back to biblical times. Many people in modern society, however, seek to deny the existence of this life-style and the group of individuals who pursue it. Society does not sanction such relationships and rarely understands them. The widespread belief that these relationships are short-lived and based only on sex makes it difficult for most people to acknowledge the affectional bond that can exist between two men. Many states legally prohibit sexual expression of this love. Although many action-oriented groups (Gay Liberation, Queer Nation, etc.) have lobbied for the rights of homosexuals and have attempted to change public opinion, societal and professional attitudes, including those of social workers, remain firmly entrenched.

Society offers little opportunity for the overt expression of grief and bereavement in general, and even less opportunity for gay men. Even as gay men grieve, they are subject to homophobia. Stigma is often attached to any survivor who has lost a significant other. Parkes (1972) characterizes this stigma as a change in attitude that takes place in society when a person dies. Every widow discovers that people who were previously friendly and approachable become embarrassed and strained in her presence.

Goffman (1963) defines stigma as the situation of the individual who is disqualified from full social acceptance. He outlines three categories of stigma, and includes homosexuality when he refers to blemishes of individual characteristics. Because society conditions its members to feel apprehensive toward those who lead alternative life-styles, it is difficult for gay men to receive support while they mourn their losses. The absence of societal sanction for intimate, same-sex relationships contributes to the prolongation of the grieving process.

Researchers recognize a need to include nonkin relationships in studies of grief. As early as 1974, Folta and Deck noted: "While all of these studies tell us that grief is a normal phenomenon, the intensity of which corresponds to the closeness of the relationship with the deceased, they fail to take the (i.e., friendship) into account. The underlying assumption is that "closeness of relationship" exists only among spouses and/or immediate kin" (239). Similarly, Raphael (1983), in her comprehensive review of grief reactions, considers that "there may be other dyadic partnership relationships in adult life that show patterns similar to conjugal ones, among them the young couple intensely, even secretly in love; the de facto relationship, the extra-marital relationship and the homosexual couple" (227).

Until recently, few researchers have studied the phenomenon of grief and bereavement among male homosexuals (Weinbach 1989; Klein & Fletcher 1986; Siegal & Hoefer 1981). There appears to be increased tolerance and recognition for the needs of gay survivors whose partners become ill with AIDS, experience the ravages of the disease and die. Kimmel (1978), writing before the advent of the AIDS crisis, notes some of the conflicts experienced by gay men during their lovers' illnesses. He wrote of an older gay man who told his sibling about losing his lover of forty years. When his partner became ill he could not risk asking for time off from work for fear of disclosing the nature of the relationship to his employer.

With their experience of repeated loss, gay survivors often have to struggle against being identified as blameworthy persons. Siegal and Hoefer (1981) highlight problems such as hostility from families and exclusion from the planning of funeral arrangements, or even from the service itself. Unless relatives exhibit an unusual level of acceptance, inheritance arrangements are problematic for most homosexual survivors. Church officials conducting services may also convey their own negative feelings.

Parkes (1972) states that there is considerable evidence to suggest that bereavement is a major hazard to the health of the surviving spouse or relative. Unresolved relationship issues often emerge. The grieving homosexual may experience intolerance from people at work who are unaware that their co-worker is grieving the loss of his life partner, rather than merely the loss of a friend. This lack of support and acknowledgment further complicates grief.

Clearly, the bereaved homosexual is at risk of being overwhelmed by social pressures. As a result, he may not successfully work through the grief toward reintegration into his community or social group. In a study of recently bereaved widows, Raphael (1984) found that a combination of factors inhibit normal healthy grief. These factors, which can apply to homosexuals who are grieving, include: traumatic circumstances surrounding the death; the widow perceives her (his) social network as nonsupportive; a pathological marital relationship existed (including marked dependence or ambivalence); another crisis occurs concurrently (multiple deaths). It is obvious that any or all of these factors may predispose the surviving homosexual partner to many psychological difficulties that would inhibit normal healthy grief.

Abnormal grief reactions may be similarly experienced by clinicians. Failure to resolve painful feelings is often maintained by avoidance of all things that provoke grief. Ramsey and De Groot (1984) associate abnormal grief with a phobic reaction that manifests itself in high levels of anxiety and avoidance of the situations in which anxiety is experienced. Hodgkinson (1982) states that in all cases the formulation is basically the same, that is, a failure at some level to acknowledge and accept the death and relinquish the deceased. The person denies the death by inhibiting grief or perpetuates expressed grief as a continued link with the dead person.

There is little doubt that a major resource for coping with grief is the availability of social support networks, which provide comfort and share the loss. Homosexual men are forced to suppress their grief processes if there is an absence of supports. Their potential sources of support are limited to relatives or friends who knew of the relationship and can be trusted. Close friends and relatives who knew of the relationship, but were overtly or tacitly disapproving, may recognize the extent of the loss. Their previous communications of disapproval of the relationship may preclude their being viewed as a potential source of help. They may be "secretly" happy that the relationship has been terminated, or offer the unhelpful cliche that "you have to get on with your life." Bereaved persons and researchers in thanatology have consistently found this response to be harmful to the grieving process (Parkes 1980; Davidowitz & Myreck 1984).

RECOVERING AFTER THE DEATH

Recovering from the devastation of losing one's lover to AIDS is a long and complex process. Jackson (1979) describes grief as a silent, knifelike terror and sadness that comes a hundred times a day, when you start to speak to someone who is no longer there. Doka (1987) claims that bereavement can be complicated in traditional relationships and intensified in nontraditional ones, because resources for resolving grief are often limited, formal and informal systems may be unavailable, and religion (which may be disapproving of homosexuality) and rituals may constrain rather than facilitate grief.

Tension between a widow and her husband's family is classic in both professional and popular literature. The vulnerability of the surviving gay spouse, who has neither legal family status nor a socially sanctioned position as the true partner of his lover, makes his a unique situation (Geis, Fuller & Rush 1986). This is further complicated by fears of his own mortality, shared fears of contagion and a resurgence of internalized homophobia (Paradis 1990), as illustrated in the following case:

Henry, a thirty-six-year-old Jewish homosexual, was referred to the Employee Assistance Program (EAP) at his place of work by the director of personnel. He had risen through the ranks from a lab technician to supervisor at a reputable suburban hospital. Henry was well liked and respected in his position. He did not disclose his homosexuality since AIDS was a "disturbing illness" when he was hired ten years ago. He lived with a number of men prior to his last relationship of eight and a half years with Paul. Neither man disclosed his gay life-style to his family or employer. Paul died one year ago and Henry continued to convey to his co-workers his "happy-go-lucky self." It was not until the suicide attempt in the lab that his need for help surfaced.

During his first visit to the EAP office, the social worker conveyed interest and concern as Henry painfully described his feelings of intense shame, guilt, humiliation and helplessness in "letting go." He was able to express his profound feelings of despair, isolation and lack of comfort since Paul's death. He cried, saying he never asked for help and felt that killing himself would be a simple solution to stop the pain.

After assessing Henry's emotional state, the practitioner felt Henry's attitude toward self and life were hopeful. His social supports were explored. Henry had a number of gay friends to whom he was close, but did not want to burden them with his problems. The worker sensitively explored Henry's feelings of burden, and it became evident that he feared rejection. He felt he would begin to reach out by calling his sister and spending the next few days with her, since she knew of his life-style and Paul's death. Henry expressed relief in talking about Paul and his worries and said he did not feel judged by the worker. He agreed to return to the worker the next day.

The worker met with Henry on a weekly basis over an eighteen month period. They used the time to help identify and sort out Henry's feelings about himself and to gain some alternatives to his feeling abandoned. Henry also began to understand his guilt as a survivor and why he was so overwhelmed and felt there was "no way out." As he began to feel more confident, he started to spend more time with his friends. He also joked about "taking off his mask at work." The social worker pursued this with him and helped him to trust himself more and learn new ways of coping and attending to his day-to-day needs. In the last session, Henry said he believed that each of us can affect our own life and death, through our attitudes toward ourselves and others. "I have come to realize that my pleasures, expectations and priorities have changed since Paul's death. I feel people will be there for me if I let them know even when I am feeling lonely."

Doka (1987) states that the availability of social supports is a factor that facilitates bereavement. Yet gay partners like Henry are often hesitant or unable to count on the support of their biological families, their friends or social institutions. Friends may push the surviving lover through the bereavement process because they are emotionally drained or undergoing their own bereavement overload (Murphy & Perry 1988; Barrows & Halgin 1988). For example, friends may prematurely try to get the bereaved to attend parties and to develop new romantic interests.

The nature of the difference between loss of a spouse and loss of a gay

partner, and the generalizability of knowledge on conjugal loss to the experiences of gay men, are areas not sufficiently researched (Martin 1988). In
a 1985 study of 745 gay men in New York City, Martin found that 27% had
experienced the death of at least one lover or close friend to AIDS, and one-
third of these had had multiple losses. He saw a direct relationship between
the number of bereavements and symptoms of traumatic stress response,
sleep problems, demoralization, sedative use, recreational drug use and the
use of psychological services. Martin raised a concern about the health of
those gay men who are HIV-positive given the possible immunologic deficits
that are known to follow bereavement.

Members of an AIDS-related bereavement group following the death of
a partner reported a range of intense feelings—sadness, sorrow, isolation,
loneliness and anger. They experienced waves of emotions, from numbness,
relief and disorientation to fear. Sometimes they would cry for no apparent
reason, and other times they felt as if they were falling apart. Some said
they felt progressions of feelings such as numbness, momentary upset, pro-
ductivity, especially at work, followed by being energized with anger.

This range of emotions is demonstrated in the following case of Jim, a
forty-nine-year old African-American:

Jim began the session by telling the therapist that he was in a relationship of twelve
years when he met Bill and fell head over heels in love. Jim tried to stay with his
lover, Steve, but found it impossible to do so. After an acrimonious separation, he
and Bill began a live-in relationship. He described it as one of the most satisfying
experiences of his life. They shared mutual interests in square dancing, theatre,
activities with gay friends and associates in their respective employments.

"Six months after the relationship began I learned that Steve was diagnosed with
AIDS. I felt so guilty, knowing I should be there to care for him. Within weeks,
Bill was diagnosed HIV-positive and within ten months he too had full-blown AIDS."
Jim told of the ravages of the illness on Bill, the dissatisfying care during his many
hospitalizations, and Jim's efforts to make the last months of his lover's life as full
and comfortable as possible. "My two sisters and brother knew Bill and were sources
of support for both of us. They not only visited Bill in the hospital but helped me
with his funeral arrangements. After Bill's death, I feel I should have done more. I
met a friend at a gay choral group and he suggested I talk to you about my excruciating
pain." The worker acknowledged Jim's feelings of guilt at leaving Steve and his anger
and disappointment in being alone. They talked about the difficulties of losing people
that we love and feelings of being a survivor. Jim cried profusely, and said he had
not cried since the funeral. "I stay in the apartment and look at home movies to quiet
my loneliness. It's hard to imagine being with my friends or becoming involved with
anyone, although I long for a warm hug."

Over a period of two years, Jim brought in a scrapbook that he put together of
memorable times with both Bill and Steve. He felt it was a way of keeping the good
times alive. "This makes me feel less angry and sad because I feel less helpless. I still
feel a lot of guilt and sometimes have to work hard when I hear the voice say, you

should have died instead of them. I know that God did not want it that way and it makes me feel good to say this to you and also to my sisters and brother."

Jim's case illustrates aspects of grief and also a sense of having to continue with life. Even when the will to live may seem lost, involvement with life is not easily relinquished when the worker can focus on thoughts and feelings that seem to strengthen the client's hope of getting better, and his trust in life and love, which draw him again into the present and future. For gay survivors like Jim, an acknowledgment of completing unfinished business related to the deceased lover and friend is essential. This process can both emancipate and provide a perspective on the lover's survivorship and his unique shared history with his deceased partner.

Guilt and Other Psychological Reactions

Guilt is an important aspect of adverse grief responses and seems to play a large part in most losses. Geis, Fuller and Rush (1986) report on the guilt and responsibility that homosexual partners feel when their lover dies of AIDS. Early in the bereavement process, the surviving lover may cry in anguish or be numbed and nonresponsive. He may engage in frantic activity, trying desperately to shut out or undo the enormity of what has happened. Waves of anger and remorse, self-blame for not always realizing how very ill their lover was and guilt for having met their own needs during their lover's illness are some of the concerns voiced by respondents. For gay men the concern expressed in the "if only" type of guilt may be exacerbated by guilt about their sexual orientation. The guilt can be over things said and done, or over acts of omission. A sense of unfinished business is often brought to one's awareness by death. Deep feelings of thwarted hopes, outrage at the uncontrollable poor timing and the unavoidable sense of injustice that accompanies this type of death are experienced by the surviving lover.

Common among gay survivors is the feeling that they contributed to their lover's death. Many come to this conclusion because they had not persuaded the lover to obtain care earlier. Some may also be HIV-positive and asymptomatic—perhaps the actual source of their partner's infection. On the other hand, some feel guilty at having persuaded their lover to go through the pain, tests, nausea and humiliating isolation that became part of their treatment. The survivor is especially vulnerable to feelings that he and his partner may have been punished for their behaviors. Fear, guilt and resentment of being a survivor is often felt.

If the bereaved believes—rightly or wrongly—that his actions contributed to the death, then it may be even more difficult to resolve the loss. This may appear in survival themes such as numbing, in absent or delayed grief or in extreme guilt. Because of the horror of some AIDS deaths, the death is likely to be linked, consciously or unconsciously, in the lover's mind to his own destructive fantasies and particularly to any violent feelings or thoughts he ever had toward the deceased person. In his fantasy the survivor's ambivalence about the deceased person seems to have contributed to the death, bringing further guilt and despair to punish the survivor for remaining alive.

The case of Jim presented earlier vividly reflects the guilt experienced by gay men, which influences their grief work:

As Jim talked to his therapist, he questioned why Bill died when he was allowed to continue living. He described himself as much less worthy, having fewer ambitions and talents, and considerably less to live for. He raved about the success Bill would have been in the movie industry, how physically attractive and vital he was and how charming he was with friends and relatives. When asked whether his friends felt the same way, he retorted that they really did not know what a cad he (Jim) was. When the worker wondered what he meant, he talked about feeling punished for abandoning his first lover, Steve, as precipitously as he had, at a time when he was most needed. Jim talked about how considerate and understanding Steve was and revealed that he died within months of Bill's death. Jim felt that although Bill's and his love was special, it could not last because Jim was being punished for his callous behavior.

The worker explored Jim's sense of himself as quite unrealistic. His maladaptive defenses were used to protect his unrealistic perception of himself. His difficulty stemmed from early childhood when he did not derive a realistic sense of being cared about and valued. The worker, being both encouraging and empathic, attempted to help Jim identify those patterns that were self-defeating and to engage him in modifying them. This work helped Jim understand his earlier experiences and allowed him to explore his guilt. After expressing his anger he appeared less depressed. With support and understanding he emerged as being less harsh on himself.

Using insight-oriented techniques, as in Jim's case, helps correct earlier experiences that clients undergo in the present, which can be exacerbated by loss or death. A lover's death, particularly if it is a suicide, may restimulate old self-doubts, negative feelings, and insecurities about being gay. The inability to grieve and to be part of the "letting go" of a significant other may delay resolution of feelings and result in other psychological reactions.

One gay survivor described to his therapist dreams, recurring images and thoughts of his lover returning and waiting for him at their favorite restaurant. When the worker explored his feelings of loneliness, the survivor recognized that this behavior was a temporary comfort, and a way to cope with the loss. "It keeps me 'alive,' but it has its limits." He laughingly said that he had arranged his first date following his loss at this restaurant, thinking it would help him deal with the feelings he had kept on hold.

Some lovers report being filled with guilt for having left their lovers under the stress of the dying process, and for feeling the need to protect themselves. This abandonment of the relationship compounded feelings of intense guilt. Some partners were unable to withstand the emotional tension incurred during the dying process and, out of terror and anger, forced their lover to leave. Some lovers also were chased from the scene of the illness by families who were determined to do their own caregiving and who disapproved of their relative's life-style and his gay partner.

There was an outpouring of frustration by one survivor who said he and his partner used safe-sex precautions, but still discovered that his lover had AIDS. The possibility of infection creates barriers to future intimacy. Another survivor said he viewed his fears as irrational since he was monogamous, but was preoccupied with the possibility of infection. This preoccupation leads survivors to regard their own relatively minor medical symptoms as ominous. Often the bonds are strong enough to sustain the partnership, but anger is paramount as the survivor feels threatened by the death of his lover and the possibility of being infected. The fear of developing the disease is both acute and very painful. In view of our current knowledge of the routes of transmission, the fear is painfully realistic.

In cases where the survivor cares for a lover during the dying process, relief and guilt are often expressed after the death. The combination of guilt and relief is stimulated by gratitude that the lover is no longer suffering, and that the responsibility and emotional demands of caregiving are over. It is not unusual for a lover to experience resentment over feeling compelled to remain in a relationship with a dying partner out of moral obligation. The emotional toll and feelings of withdrawal and isolation are a lot to endure. This degree of ambivalence is not as evident in more stable and open relationships. Any ambivalence expressed is usually more related to stressful events prior to HIV infection and AIDS.

A number of survivors expressed anger at the deceased lover for deserting them, leaving the survivor alone to cope with the emotionally painful and often frustrating process of making burial arrangements, obtaining death certificates and settling estates. Anger was often directed, sometimes inappropriately, at the health care system, doctors, nurses and other hospital personnel for their poor communication and lack of empathy. In addition, there was anger during discussions with families of the deceased concerning mutual properties. Some partners felt they had no legal rights to apartments and household properties they had purchased jointly.

Men in our society are expected to suppress their urge to cry. The worker can anticipate typical conflicts for the survivor over whether or not to publicly acknowledge the relationship. By withholding emotions, the survivor may say he is just a friend of the deceased. When concealing the truth about sexuality, many gay people attempt to pass off their intimate relationships as an arrangement between roommates or friends. As a result of this hiding of feelings and truths, the depth of emotional pain during the grieving process may be intensified, self-esteem further damaged and guilt feelings channeled into self-destructive behavior. Memories can become a painful reminder of loneliness when they cannot be shared with others. One respondent felt his greatest release was when he met a former friend and "sobbed like a baby" as they reminisced about shared experiences. Although crying as an expression of feelings is foreign to many men, the ability to let go in a safe place often is a helpful release.

PERSONAL VULNERABILITY

The loss and sense of aloneness felt after the death of a partner can be magnified by a gay man's fear that other men will not want to become involved with him. The grieving partner will need support when he initiates sexual and romantic involvement, particularly if he does experience the anticipated rejection and fear of others. Some men have no intimate physical contact with others for extended periods after the death of their lover. Many avoid these potentially satisfying contacts out of an irrational fear that they may contaminate someone else. AIDS-induced fears, such as the fear of being a carrier or the fear of having contracted AIDS from their deceased partner, need to be expressed and dealt with. According to Klein and Fletcher (1986), this fear of AIDS in the gay community has a tremendous impact on the survivor's reentry into a social environment and his ability to meet new partners. For the older gay male especially, it is traumatic enough to search for a fitting companion in a youth-oriented subculture without added fears of acquiring or transmitting a terminal disease.

As Simos (1986) points out, "There is a temptation of the bereaved to seek premature replacement objects as a defense against the pain of grief" (247). Becoming involved in new relationships, cruising the bars and discos and abusing alcohol or drugs can be forms of resistance to exploring the impact of the loss of a lover. To prevent future difficulties in interpersonal relationships, loss must be worked through rather than denied. Worden (1982) states that verbal expression of ambivalence and anger at having to continue on alone must be encouraged.

Preoccupation with their health was found in newly bereaved gay men (Murphy & Perry 1988; Oerlemans-Bunn 1988). These authors state that physical symptoms of stress are found with all significant losses, but that gay men whose lovers have died of AIDS are at higher risk than others of contracting HIV infection because bereavement reduces resistance to infections. AIDS survivors also fear that they will become ill and not have anyone to care for them as they cared for their lovers. These worries can be overwhelming. Consequently, many wish to escape into death, and some are at risk for suicide.

Emotional problems associated with concealment of a socially stigmatized life-style may be heightened during the mourning process, unless significant others exhibit a level of acceptance. If the survivor has not disclosed his homosexual relationship or his lover's death from AIDS to family, friends or workmates, the resulting isolation and self-protection will add significantly to the emotional assault on his well-being. The survivor will not be able to explain adequately any resulting changes in his behavior and functioning. The isolation will be permeated by a fear of further losses—loss of job, friendships or family ties. Ventilation of the surviving lover's fear, frustration and grief with a supportive person or therapist is crucial.

ROLE OF FAMILY AND FRIENDS

Certain rituals and customs are undertaken to help survivors process the loss of loved ones. Planning and participation in funeral rites are aids in adjusting to grief (Doka 1987). Supportive family and friends are likely to rally around; the bereaved lover can commence the painful process of mourning, and can say good-bye. Some lovers feel acknowledged and fully participate in the funeral service, the eulogies and the death notices.

In nontraditional relationships, survivors lose a significant role when the partner dies, and there is no defined role (as in grieving widow) for them to assume. In cases in which the relationship is secret, there naturally is no recognition of grief. The relatives of the deceased person, especially those who were not aware of his life-style, may question or be suspicious of the gay survivor if he attends a memorial service or funeral as a final act of love. The surviving lover or friend may not be able to attend the funeral service for numerous reasons, including fear of confirming rumors or creating suspicion.

Doka (1987) and Murphy and Perry (1988) found that homosexual lovers were often excluded from the planning process and from participation in or recognition at funerals, wakes or memorial services. In some ways, it is as if the relationship never existed. If gay survivors attend the services, they must carefully guard their grief. Their very presence may lead to resentment and hostile comments from those who knew of or suspected the relationship. A visit by the gay survivor to his deceased lover's family may create an even more difficult situation, compounding feelings of guilt, anger or discomfort.

The following case demonstrates the complexity of grief in relationships that are not recognized:

After a brief, intense sexual relationship, Ron and Bob became very good friends. Their friendship was special to both of them and they repeatedly acknowledged not ever having such a meaningful relationship with another male. They talked frequently by phone, met with some regularity for drinks or dinner, and occasionally went cruising together. They confided and kept each other informed of their successes or failures in establishing intimate contacts.

Ron was divorced, the father of two children and an accomplished professional. Bob was also the father of two children and a professional but was currently married. Although they talked about Bob's experiences in the marriage and as a father, their relationship was a secret from his family.

During one of their routine phone calls, Bob informed his friend that he was having some difficulties with a bronchial condition and intractable diarrhea. After a week of such complaints he indicated that he was going to see his physician, but did not seem worried. The next phone call to Ron was from the hospital, with the information that Bob had been diagnosed as HIV-positive. They talked about when Ron could pay a visit and agreed that within a week, when his wife had developed a routine for her visits, arrangements could be made.

When Ron did not hear from his friend after seven days, he called the hospital to learn that the number he had been given was disconnected. He immediately called Bob's work number and was told by a secretary that Bob had died over the weekend. Ron was devastated and felt totally unconnected, confused and frustrated. He found himself frantically searching the obituary columns to find out whether a public funeral had been announced, since he could not call the family's home to inquire. Since his search was unsuccessful, Ron was left to cope with his grief, which was complicated by the intense bonding he had shared with Bob, the secret aspects of their relationship and the lack of an opportunity to say good-bye.

After several weeks, Ron returned to the therapist he had seen when he was going through his divorce. He used the opportunity to cry and rage at such an unfortunate and precipitous ending of his relationship with Bob. The therapist consoled him and helped him work through and resolve his intense grief. He told the therapist of returning to many of the places he and Bob frequented, of trying to relive some of the experiences they had shared and of how incomplete he felt. The therapist continued to be supportive of Ron, using their time together to review his life with Bob and acknowledging the difficulty Ron was experiencing in lacking public recognition of his grief. They spoke about closure and finding an opportunity to visit the graveside or undertake a ritual that he and Bob would enjoy and using the solitary process to let go.

Ron's case is a good example of grief, complicated by secrecy. Had his relationship with Bob been publicly acknowledged, he would have been able to see his friend prior to the latter's death, to have talked about their relationship and find some level of comfort in the numerous meaningful experiences they had shared. This anticipatory process would have significantly reduced the extent and difficulty of the mourning. Participating in the funeral services would have provided closure, despite the normal anguish and pain of mourning. Absent from these opportunities, Ron searched, unsuccessfully, for meaning of his friend's death by returning to their previous haunts.

The sensitivity of his therapist, while allowing and encouraging him to mourn outwardly, is demonstrated most clearly by her encouraging him to engage in a ritual, posthumously shared with Bob, which acknowledges the significance of the relationship and gives closure that permits Ron to move on.

SOCIAL SUPPORTS

Social support is the assistance or activities through which people help others satisfy their needs and cope with problems when they arise. Since grief can disable a bereaved person emotionally, physically and behaviorally, assistance is needed from others. Grievers benefit from emotional support or from care, love, trust and empathy from others. Instrumental support, in the form of doing things for the griever, is also helpful. Taking physical care of the survivor or undertaking routine tasks for him, such as paying bills, frees up the bereaved person's energy for dealing with grief.

Another form of support that gay grievers find useful may be termed appraisal support. This support consists of information that the survivor may use for self-evaluation or social comparison. Gay grievers find solace in knowing that their grief is not unique, and that feelings of self-doubt, anguish and a wish to die are similar to what other bereaved persons experience. Practitioners need to consider which forms of support are the responsibility of nonprofessionals—significant individuals in the griever's environment—and which forms of support professionals should provide.

While death often creates a sense of chaos, people strive to reinstate order and to understand and control their life circumstances. Reducing uncertainty and enhancing control are central functions of social support (Albrecht & Adelman 1987). According to Parkes (1980), one of the critical factors in facilitating bereavement is the presence of social supports. Although the extent and nature of social supports available to gay men whose lovers have died from AIDS vary, and the men's evaluation of the effectiveness of these supports change over time, the social network functions as the mainstay of support, self-expression and resources during a time of loss.

Active listening to the distress of the gay survivor is a major component of social support. It is often through a stream of talk that the bereaved individual derives a sense of the coherence of troubling life circumstances. Friends are often a major source of this sort of support. They can become a burden, however, when they are unable or unwilling to provide the help a survivor needs (Pearlin, Semple & Turner 1988).

The importance of emotional support has been demonstrated by Zich and Temoshok (1987). They examined the degree of support available to persons with AIDS using measures of social support, hardiness and physical and psychological distress. Measures of support included four major categories of helping: (1) emotionally sustaining behaviors (for example, having someone to talk to); (2) problem-solving behaviors (having someone offer suggestions); (3) indirect personal influence (for example, having someone convey a willingness to help); and (4) environmental action (having someone intervene to reduce environmental stress). The authors found that, in comparison to problem-solving help, emotionally sustaining forms of help were viewed as more desirable, more available, more often used and more helpful when used.

Given the stigma associated with formal therapeutic assistance, it may be that voluntary informal support from family and friends is more effective in bolstering self-esteem and in helping the bereaved lover cope with the death. Reaffirmation of intrinsic qualities and support of the individual's coping response are vital to restoring a sense of self-worth. The likelihood of going to the lover's family is very rare (Siegal and Hoefer, 1981). While some families are accepting, many are not, leading to bitter arguments over funeral arrangements, financial settlements and disposal of possessions (Geis, Fuller & Rush 1986; Greif & Porembski 1988; Murphy & Perry 1988).

Informal social support networks can have a buffering effect that aids the bereaved person in coping with the death. Psychological well-being is enhanced by the knowledge that one can depend on others in a time of need. In addition to buffering against the crisis of death, informal networks often compensate for the assistance that would otherwise be provided formally by professionals.

Gay men who have lost their lover to AIDS often lack adequate social supports (Barrows & Halgin 1988; Doka 1987; Murphy & Perry 1988; Oerlemans-Bunn 1988; Pearlin, Semple & Turner 1988). Isolation, unresolved stress and lack of adequate social supports, as described by Gonsiorek (1982), play a significant role in perpetuating depression among bereaved homosexuals. The lack of resources designed for gay people creates a difficult situation for the bereaved person. When one is gay and lives in a community where homosexuality is not considered acceptable, where does one seek solace? Gay men cannot go to a priest or rabbi because homosexuals are considered sinners. Gay men may not be able to go to a doctor, lawyer or work supervisor for fear of exposure, loss of a job or status in the community. Most gay men cannot expect support from their families for fear of rejection.

Emotional support many not alleviate the bereaved homosexual's sense of hopelessness and depression. Zich and Temoshok (1987) find significant negative correlations between hopelessness or depression and the perceived availability of social support. They conclude that highly needy persons may drain the emotional resources of others and may thus receive less social support. People back away from others in trouble. In this instance, there is also guilt by association. People experiencing depression may also be less likely to perceive the availability and usefulness of social support because they are unable to reciprocate adequately. Furthermore, depressed people tend to have low self-esteem, to be highly self-focussed under negative circumstances and to be more pessimistic than those who are not depressed.

The more dependent the survivor has been in the relationship, the more likely it is that the after-effects of the shock will be acute and long-lasting. If the gay survivor can reach out to other gay persons and transform feelings of loss, anger, guilt and loneliness into feelings of self-regard and self-interest, it will be easier for him to be validated in his social identity.

Precipitous moves tend to be made when support systems are weak and survivors have no one to whom they can turn (Simos 1986). If there is not even a minimal social network, the survivor is more likely to move, escape or embark upon a major life change, often with disastrous consequences, rather than cope with the added stresses (Siegal & Hoefer 1981). If the gay survivor shows evidence of having an impulsive or cyclothymic personality, he is more likely to become suicidal. Early signs of self-destructive behavior should be monitored by professionals and there should be ongoing assessment of risk or sudden change of mood.

Role of Support Groups

Survivors need to connect to a support system. One potent support system that is often underutilized is the support group. Membership in support groups is critical, given the fact that grievers find people helpful in different ways depending where they are in the grieving process. The possibility of hope and strength that is provided in a group is basic to coping with grief.

A major function of self-help groups is to provide a pool of comparable others from whose experiences judgments about oneself can be derived. Such bereavement groups enable the people to make upward comparisons (comparing themselves with those who are better off), horizontal comparisons (comparing themselves with those whose circumstances are seen as similar) and downward comparisons (comparing themselves with those who are worse off). Participants in such groups can derive a sense of shared fate with similar others ("I'm not in this alone"), and can compare their present situation with potentially worse alternatives ("Things could be worse") (Wills 1987). As grievers become helpers, the two-way exchange reduces feelings of dependency. This role shift is critical to sustaining a sense of control and active participation in the course of grieving.

Participation in support groups was acknowledged by a number of gay respondents as critical to their coping with the death of their lover. Some were involved in a support group during the caregiving period, and one member poignantly stated that with AIDS your spirits are continually getting tested and hope is pitted against hopelessness . . . yet, it is those around you who know what you are experiencing and give you reasons to go on. Support groups are also instrumental in assisting surviving partners to rebuild their self-concept and to manage a daily life that is no longer predicated on a merged identity or a caregiving role. For many the shift from complete immersion in helping their lover to sudden isolation brings anticipated but nonetheless disjunctive role changes. The emotional support provided by group members helps gay survivors avoid self-blame and guilt and provides a place for them to share information, gain mastery and discuss difficult issues such as sexuality and fear of infection.

Leon is an example of a gay survivor whose experience in a support group minimized his isolation. In the support group, Leon spoke about his feelings.

As Ken lay dying from AIDS, Leon, who was Ken's lifetime companion, felt angry and confused about his loss and Ken's impending death. Some of the friends he shared with Ken tried to help him by talking to him during the week, joining him in visits to the hospital and sharing in the responsibilities of physical care. Weekly dinners continued on Wednesday nights. Leon reported that without the group, he probably would have attempted suicide to escape the pain.

When Ken died, Leon was inconsolable. Unlike his friends he projected a sense of stoicism and strength, refusing to cry or "break down." He appeared to be in full charge of himself, causing his friends to comment about how well he was coping with Ken's death. Don, the self-appointed manager of the weekly supper group, learned that Leon was visiting Ken's grave daily. Don felt that this was inappropriate and suggested that Leon join a bereavement group at the Gay Men's Health Crisis Center. Reluctantly, Leon agreed and began attending a weekly support group.

He was surprised to meet men like himself who had lost friends or lifetime companions to AIDS. Initially, Leon thought the revelations of the members were morbid and served no purpose. He felt it would be better to bury and forget rather than revive memories of Ken. When he felt pressure from the group to recall what he and Ken liked to do, how they met and how their friendship grew, he was surprised how relieved he felt. He gained an understanding of what had developed between Ken and himself and of what he had lost as a consequence of Ken's death. Leon also learned that while he could not replace that friendship, he could become aware of his capacity to develop other meaningful relationships.

Several months later, when talking to Don, Leon found himself telling about how sensitive and skillful the group leader was and how he was so resistant in exploring his loss. Leon felt a release of powerful emotions by group members that he could identify with and found a place where he felt safe and less isolated. The encouragement and support of men with common feelings and experiences was liberating and reduced Leon's feeling of guilt, depression, anxiety and helplessness, all common feelings of grief.

Bereavement groups for gay survivors help them grieve not only for their dead and dying friends but also for a way of life that is gone and may never come again. The consolation of intimate contact that support groups provide is both productive and powerful in the grieving process. To associate with people who share the same problem, predicament or life situation and who unite for the purpose of mutual support is empowering.

"MOVING ON"

For most bereaved people, to keep going after the painful life changes caused by death is the most difficult task of all. When a lover dies, the loss plunges the bereaved person into a world where the known and habitual structures of daily life disappear into a world of confusion, disorganization and anxiety. A new order has to be constructed. The bereaved lover begins to find new ways of interacting with others as well as of reconciling the fragmentation of his personal identity with everyday realities.

Accepting that the lover is dead and is never coming back begins healing the wounds of loss. Reassurance that a wide range of feelings and thoughts is a normal part of grieving helps to facilitate the mourning. First anniversaries of the lover's death, his birthday and holidays enjoyed together are remembered and strong feelings are acknowledged. This feeling was reflected in one group member's statement: "It was difficult to get through the firsts and I found one of the hardest times to be alone was on my birthday when we would go to Fire Island and have a bash."

For some, there are practical problems to deal with, such as having bank accounts, credit cards and medical insurance changed to reflect the lover's death. For others, the shift in roles has to do with the transition of living alone and learning to cook for one. As one group member noted: "The hardest time for me was sitting down and eating my first dinner alone, which was about two months after Ted died. The next few days, I invited someone to dinner every night, just to have someone at the table."

Some lovers have difficulty reintegrating themselves into the gay male community, while others become involved in gay or AIDS-related service or political organizations. For still others, the experience of death leaves them with an existential detachment and a sense that things are transitory and that life is to be lived now.

Lindemann (1944) notes that "a needed transition to looking ahead eventually arises, and signals a willingness to deal with the task of emancipation from bondage to the deceased." A shift to living in the absence of the dead lover entails a good deal of adaptation. Seeking to assume or reassign roles, as well as freeing oneself from some that are replaceable, not wanted or needed in the lover's absence, is a long process.

Moving into a new social scene and learning to mix and mingle and meet people is difficult for many reasons. Facing people in the gay community, which has been consumed by AIDS, and where despair evokes fear, is distinctly difficult for a single, bereaved homosexual as he pursues a new long-term love relationship.

Grief work begins with mourning the deceased. The amount of time to work through grief can vary greatly, especially in AIDS epicenters, where multiple losses are common. Significant dates, events, sights, music and places can provide important opportunities and even rituals for working through the loss of a lover or friend.

IMPLICATIONS FOR PRACTITIONERS

When a gay partner dies of AIDS, many complex reactions must be faced. In regard to bereavement, the gay survivor faces a double stigma. Not only must the survivor cope with the death of his lover, but often he must reveal himself as a gay man. Survivors of gay lovers and friends constitute a relatively new population of grievers for whom there are few guidelines for care, few experts and few resources to be consulted. These deaths are often particularly untimely, and occur under difficult and sometimes tragic circumstances. It is always felt that they should not have happened. Not only do gay men have to cope with the grief and guilt of survivorship, but they experience the onslaught of multiple deaths among friends and the loss of total communities.

A practitioner who chooses to work with gay clients should be aware of her or his conscious or unconscious thoughts, attitudes and responses to gay life-styles. Throughout the process of grieving the clinician can help bereaved gay men let go of an intimate, significant other and develop positive, specific changes in their personal growth and social interactions. Awareness of the client's reactions to the stigma of being gay and to the stigma of being a mourner is essential for the clinician in order to help the griever understand these feelings. The practitioner should explore specific grief reactions with gay men and recognize survivor guilt feelings as part of the struggle to deal with multiple losses. In treating adverse grief reactions, the clinician should be aware of the role that denial plays in response to an overwhelming amount of grief. Denial can have an adaptive function in one's life, and the worker must be cautious how she/he approaches the denial.

The clinician can explore specific, individualized strategies or rituals to acknowledge anniversaries or events, which can enhance the mourning process. Friends and family can be included to share in the recognition of the lover's death and the survivor's loss. Resolution of grief will be accompanied by less guilt, greater self-esteem and stronger coping mechanisms to meet ongoing life challenges. More than anything, the gay survivor needs help in rebuilding his life without his partner.

In treatment, an examination of the redemptive irony of loss is of particular importance. Because AIDS affects large numbers of homosexuals who may perceive their life-styles as socially unacceptable to others, it may be difficult for surviving partners to find meaning in their misfortune or to express their feelings to others. This perceived stigma may force them to be silent about the death to others who do not share their life-style. Encouraging the gay mourner to become involved in AIDS or gay organizations can assist in resolution of their AIDS-related grief.

Knott (1989) states that there is always gain to be found accompanying every loss. In this culture, finding that gain in not an easy task, for there are too many prohibitions against such admissions of loss. But a healing perspective comes from seeing the gains in survivorship—the strengths commanded by its psychosocial legacies, the relief, the new appreciation of what matters—death is the ultimate values clarification experience. Such awareness comes gradually over time with some tactful reframing by the clinician. It is an essential benchmark of grief resolution and of healing the wounds of loss.

As part of grief resolution, either in individual treatment, group treatment or a support group, it is important to find both a purpose and value to the relationship between the survivor and the deceased person. Often it helps to consider how the gay survivor and the deceased lover changed and developed through their relationship, by using a "life review."

CHAPTER 9

Intervening with Practitioners

As devastating as AIDS has been over the past eleven years, every projection indicates that it will become worse in all areas of the country and in all areas of the world. Increasing numbers of persons with AIDS, and their survivors, especially in poor, urban communities, are challenging social work practitioners to an extent that is unparalleled in modern times. Mental health and medical inpatient and outpatient facilities, and family and social service agencies, have been overwhelmed by the demands of providing care for people with AIDS and for their bereaved survivors.

In intervening with persons with AIDS and their bereaved survivors, practitioners are susceptible to their own grief responses of sadness, anger, guilt, depression and helplessness. As professionals constantly witness the deaths of their clients, they too become the bereaved. When death is experienced in serial fashion, without adequate processing of the multiple deaths, professionals can become subject to bereavement overload and an emotional state of "chronic mourning."

Coping with death affects many aspects of the practitioner's life. Intervening with the bereaved makes one aware of one's own losses due to death, divorce or emigration. Awareness of one's own death can hinder or deepen the work depending on the clinician's readiness to face mortality. Taboos concerning loss and death emerge in the work with concerns about homosexuality, sex, drugs and ethnic differences. Practitioners thus must acknowledge and tolerate anxiety about their own attitudes, health and issues about death.

Professionals in a variety of fields have been called upon to respond to AIDS and to work with this bereaved population. Clinicians will continue to operate mainly as institutional employees. In this capacity, they will have to face the challenge of developing their professional practice within agency systems that serve the AIDS population. Knowing what to expect in advance and being reassured that certain responses are normal can allay fears and anxieties that often engender confusion.

Professionals who intervene with people with AIDS and their survivors have to develop skills and confront the following unfamiliar stresses:

1. Illness, suffering and the multiple deaths of infants, children, adolescents and young and older adults, many of whose lives can be threatened by the severe symptoms of HIV infection without even progressing to a clinical diagnosis of AIDS.
2. Sexuality, including homosexuality, adolescent sexuality and, in some cases, sexual abuse.
3. Drug addiction among adolescents, pregnant mothers, parents and older adults.
4. Ethical quandaries such as confidentiality and issues related to birth control and abortion. (Anderson 1990, 5)

In this chapter we discuss the practitioner's personal concerns, fears and intense emotions that are evoked in the process of enabling survivors to cope. From our interviews with professionals who are in the forefront and who are experiencing a heavy emotional toll providing treatment to people with AIDS and their survivors, four areas have emerged that we will address. First, we will discuss the impact of the professional's cultural and religious values, motivation and countertransference around sex, death, difference and drug use. Second, we will consider the impact of multiple deaths on the professional. Third, we will focus on the development and maintenance of educational programs and support networks and, finally, on the causes of burnout or "compassion fatigue" and strategies in intervening with the practitioner.

The description of the professional caregiver as a survivor is appropriate in the AIDS epidemic. No similar disease has caused such widespread introspection and reexamination of how one approaches people with the disease and their bereaved significant others. In a context of fear and with a haunting reminder of the tenuousness of survival, practitioners face illness and death daily and attempt to balance their personal and professional lives. With no vaccine or cure in sight, AIDS is an exceptional challenge to professionals. Despite an extensive repertoire of therapeutic interventions that professionals bring to the treatment situation, they are not immune to prejudice fueled by fear or feelings of inadequacy and helplessness in witnessing incredible suffering.

CULTURAL AND RELIGIOUS VALUES

As is true of most problems brought to social work practitioners, AIDS challenges personal values, cultural and religious beliefs. Professionals often must confront societal disdain. For some workers a client's belief system and behaviors are in conflict with theirs, and the worker may experience discomfort and fear. How professionals have reacted in the past can provide insights about their present emotional responses and how they will grapple with these issues. The extent of awareness one has of one's own beliefs, attitudes and emotional style can clarify the issues and conflicts remaining from the past, and a perspective may be developed to respond to the ever-present stressor—death. The different effects of the stress and the range of meanings attached to AIDS inevitably affect practitioners in a variety of individualized ways.

A number of factors determine how professionals respond to this deadly, stigmatized and socially isolating disease. Psychological response to people associated with AIDS can range from acceptance to some distress to severe and lasting trauma. Transmission fears, death, social stigma, homophobia and negative attitudes toward IV drug abusers can exacerbate one's concern about what can be done on behalf of clients and how to respond professionally. Perceptions of certain people with AIDS as innocent victims (hemophiliacs, children and unknowing heterosexual partners of drug users and bisexuals), and others as guilty spreaders (homosexual and bisexual men and recreational IV drug users) must be acknowledged. Some practitioners continue to be insensitive to the needs of the bereaved survivors due to their own discomfort in discussing death.

Dunkel and Hatfield (1986) identify a range of countertransference issues that may arise for a practitioner, including: "1) fear of the unknown, 2) fear of contagion, 3) fear of dying and death, 4) denial of helplessness, 5) fear of homosexuality (homophobia), 6) overidentification, 7) anger, and 8) need for professional omnipotence" (115). Feelings about homosexuality in particular need to be faced "in order to be sure that the professional is not subtly transmitting a social bias to the surviving lover or confirming the client's own bias." Practitioners working with bereaved families of substance abusers need to identify "what they know . . . or what they do not know about the cultural lifestyles, addictive behavioral responses, and styles of defenses" (Caputo 1985, 363). By understanding the factors that jeopardize a potential or actual practice situation, clinicians can manage their countertransference feelings.

A crucial aspect of adult identity development is the integration of sexuality, including sexual orientation, into the identity. Erikson (1950) has eloquently shown that identity formation is an interactive process between the individual and society and is highly influenced by the norms and values of family and society at large. In the interplay between society and the individual, the development of gay identity differs greatly from the development of heterosexual identity. Because the norms and values of our society have been and generally remain antihomosexual, the practitioner's feelings about working with gay men, a stigmatized group, needs to be assessed. An increase in antihomosexual violence and harassment has been experienced; some people favor tattooing infected individuals and treating them as lepers by sending them off to a distant colony. What impact does this have on the practitioner?

AIDS to a great extent has forced professionals to address the propriety of adult behavior and consciously face their own perceptions and attitudes toward homosexual and bisexual men. Attitudes toward homosexuality and bisexuality vary among ethnic or religious groups even within relatively permissive societies. Within the United States, ethnic minority groups tend to be less permissive toward homosexuality. Professionals with strong ideological beliefs may not approve of the prospect of casual relationships or of a homosexual life-style. Irrational fears and prejudicial feelings about PWAs, depicting them as ugly, damaged, dirty or inferior, may interfere with treatment and result in emotional distancing, increasing the stress on the client and the worker. Although evidence of such attitudes may be less surprising among the general public (Dupree & Margo 1988), negative attitudes among professionals do exist.

Location within a given part of the country—rural, small town, or urban environment—is an important consideration in treating AIDS survivors. In small towns or rural areas of the United States where there are few openly gay men, where attitudes may be more negative and where fears or reprisals may be stronger, the professional's fear, lack of knowledge and support and dependence upon a nonaccepting environment can be of crucial import. To a large extent one cannot hide the fact of AIDS in a rural area or small town, and there is more of a chance of a person feeling ashamed or ostracized, intensifying the professional's internalized parental and societal values and prohibitions.

The combined issues of drug abuse and AIDS raise critical ethical, personal and clinical issues for practitioners. Dealing with active addiction is often frustrating; practitioners, as well as their clients, often feel a particular sense of hopelessness about AIDS and the issues surrounding substance abuse. Difficulty in working with this population emerges from the manipulative behavior on the part of addicted clients—the flattery, intrusiveness, intimidation and inflammatory remarks that can alienate and frustrate the clinician. These feelings are compounded by the mistrust and noncompliance of clients in the counseling process.

Some professionals become exceedingly uncomfortable with the prospect of passing moral judgment on the most intimate decisions made by consenting adults and on the decisions made by women about procreation, childrearing and disclosure. Most women with AIDS are poor, uneducated African-American or Hispanic women between thirteen and thirty-nine years of age. Clinicians must be attentive to their own reactions, including fear of contagion, denial and discomfort with sex, sexuality, sexual behavior change. Other issues that call for vigilance are a sense of helplessness and despair, anger and blaming the victim, blurring of ethical and professional boundaries and fear of professional inadequacy (Dilley, Pies & Helquist 1989, 247).

Conscious management of one's personal attitudes regarding other individuals' behavior is helpful in terms of something larger and something connected to the fate of the community.

Issues related to death and dying confront the professional working with bereaved AIDS survivors. There is no doubt that most clinicians are uncomfortable with discussions about death. Death can become a wall rather than a doorway. For a number of professionals, the negative connotations of death are associated substantially with feelings of rootlessness and loss of identity, loneliness and fear of going to hell. Choosing not to discuss death with survivors isolates them and deprives them of a critical experience in dealing with their own mortality and making necessary preparations.

PRACTITIONERS' MOTIVATION FOR PRACTICE WITH DEATH AND GRIEF

In the literature and in our interviews with professionals, we found a significant number of clinicians who have made a conscious decision to work with persons with AIDS and their survivors. In making this choice they were aware that death would be a significant issue in their practice, and that they would have to confront grief and bereavement. Nevertheless they chose to follow this path. Several factors preceded and influenced this decision.

Several clinicians who had unresolved losses chose to work with PWAs and, subsequently, with survivors. The level of awareness of their motivation differed among clinicians. Many participated actively and for extended periods without ever becoming aware of their principal motivation. For others, recognition of its impact and intensity came as a surprise, and with some discomfort.

Some males made the choice because of their commitment to the gay community and a recognition that AIDS and those affected were of high priority. Many had lovers, friends and acquaintances die from AIDS, and desired to make a contribution to their legacy. Other men saw it as an opportunity to "appease the powers to be"—that is, in some magical way, to forestall the likelihood that they may become ill and die from AIDS.

For women, the choice was equally varied. Many of them had relatives, friends or acquaintances who have died from AIDS, or were themselves members of groups susceptible to high-risk behavior. Other women recognized the challenge and the need for competent, dedicated professionals in this area of practice.

Few employing organizations or administrators question the motivation of practitioners who choose to work in this area. This is undoubtedly due to the need for practitioners to work in rapidly developing and expanding programs, but may also be inspired by respect for the practitioner's privacy. Nevertheless, it is important that each clinician make a conscious effort to appreciate the incentives for choosing to work with people who are dying or people who are grieving.

The reasons for being clear about one's motivation are legion. Interactions between clients and clinicians are enormously influenced by the clarity of purpose and the worker's sense of competence and commitment. Work with grievers is demanding, and is not satisfying in the typical manner of most activities in helping professions, thus increasing the potential for burnout and job dissatisfaction. Simultaneously, the work is critical to the clients, who may be at their most vulnerable stage. Clinicians, who are confused about their motivations or ambivalent about their potential for continuing in this form of practice may physically withdraw or abandon their clients. To do so would not only be detrimental to the client's well-being, but also would be professionally unethical.

Competing motivations and expectations among groups of professionals have an impact on work with clients and on the work environment. For example, gay male clinicians may question the legitimacy of straight or female practitioners working with gay PWAs and their survivors. They may conclude that clinicians who have not adopted a homosexual life-style cannot understand what it is like to be gay, to be constantly at risk of death or HIV infection or to be depreciated for behaviors considered to be natural in their life-styles. On the other hand, straight or female clinicians may envy the sense of community that gay males share and in which they can never be full participants. Similar sentiments may exist among and between African-American and Hispanic clinicians and their racially or ethnically different counterparts.

Some of these conflicts can emerge in the work with clients, as in discussions about treatment goals and techniques. They can also be expressed subtly or nonverbally. A preferred mode would be the open expression and confrontation of these professional differences. Such honest handling of differences can free clinicians to offer support and empathy to each other, necessary elements in working in the field of AIDS.

PROFESSIONAL CONCERNS

Most health care professionals are unprepared to deal with the range of issues bereaved clients encounter when their loved ones die from AIDS. A mixture of conventional, innovative and practice wisdom, as well as a compassionate response, constitute the ideal treatment approach. Intervening with survivors who are dealing with the powerful emotions associated with grief can be highly stressful for the practitioner. Despite professional education and training, perceptions on a variety of issues will be influenced both positively and negatively by the clinician's familial, cultural and socioeconomic background. Accounts from clients, media reports and limited research findings indicate that professionals share public attitudes toward contagion and discriminate against homosexual and bisexual men, IV drug users and their partners, people of color, prostitutes and adolescents who are HIV- or AIDS-infected. When the infected person dies, these discriminatory attitudes are carried over to their survivors.

Faced with the demands of treating survivors of people with AIDS, the clinician needs to draw on a variety of inner and outer resources to assist in providing human services. The literature documents the role self-appraisal plays in coping with the challenges of life. Perceptions of self-efficacy are evaluative judgments of one's own ability to manage situational demands. Bandura (1982) notes that self-perceptions of capability determine how people think and behave in stressful situations. He also demonstrates that perceptions of self-efficacy help to explain changes in coping behavior.

Those clinicians who feel they are up to the challenge, based on judgments of their own past and present problem-solving successes, may be more willing to work with people with AIDS and subsequently with their survivors. Such statements as "I don't do well with this population" or "I'm not sure my training prepared me for this" reflect, and can prompt a practitioner to become aware of, her/his counterphobic attitudes. These attitudes can diminish effectiveness in working with this population.

It is not uncommon for the professional to spend a majority of her/his time providing support and information to persons with AIDS and their survivors. Although this is an important role for health care professionals, it is not an easy task to carry out effectively. Several factors add to the complexity of the situation.

First, professionals are confronted with clients who have different levels of comprehension and varied cultural and ethnic preferences in receiving information. Sometimes providing information about child custody arrangements for the children of the deceased or the desirability of including the former lover of the deceased person in planning the funeral may empower a survivor who is poorly informed or whose powers of concentration are constricted by grief. For other clients, examination of their resistance requires confronting the nature and seriousness of their incapacitating grief, which they avoid out of fear.

No work with an individual is complete without a recognition of the client's ethnic identity, which significantly shapes one's life. Without articulating them, families manage to pass on from generation to generation beliefs, attitudes and a world view. These beliefs involve attitudes toward illness and death that are part of their ethnic and cultural identities. The professional must assess how closely the person reflects a particular heritage. While a tradition may be practiced by many people within an ethnic group, there is usually much diversity in the way that tradition is practiced. Ethnic beliefs may also be at the core of unresolved issues, and by framing them in ethnic terms, the professional encourages resolution. Rosen (1990) notes five aspects of ethnicity that can be explored when working with people around death.

These are: attitudes toward life and death; expression of pain, suffering and grief; acceptance of outside authority; expectations of family responsibility; and gender roles.

A second complicating factor in AIDS work is that information generally builds hope in people and frees them from anxiety and fear related to illness and death. Knowing the fatal outcome of the disease, clinicians feel uncomfortable at the thought of building hope in prospective survivors. Providing hope involves communicating with persons with AIDS and their survivors in ways that allow them to have positive expectations about their future even though they are confronted with highly uncertain circumstances. At this juncture in the epidemic, imparting hope is confusing to people who have received conflicting or incomplete information from the media about the disease and the course of transmission. This confusion is further compounded because AIDS disrupts virtually every aspect of a survivor's life. Everyday activities are affected, short-term and long-term goals are on hold. It is common for family members, significant others and some professionals to have lost a number of friends and loved ones to AIDS. This experience imparts the implicit message that life after the death of a loved one or associate is difficult.

Third, in addition to providing information about AIDS and correcting misconceptions, professionals need to assume responsibility for providing follow-up plans, helping with funeral arrangements, making referrals to bereavement groups and so forth. Public fears, misinformation, scapegoating, hysteria and discrimination still play a part in mobilizing limited but needed resources in responding to an epidemic of tragic proportions that will weaken if not destroy an entire generation. The greater challenge to the professional is to respond to familial and social concerns that defy easy solutions.

In recent years, the trend toward consumerism and people's growing involvement in health care decision-making have had a significant impact on the sharing of control in provider-patient relationships. The traditional medical model in which the provider is the principal decision-maker has given way to a model of interaction in which the consumer is significantly more involved in health-related issues (Schain 1980). In AIDS care, the issue of sharing control is especially important because survivors bring pronounced feelings of loss of control into ongoing health care interactions. The difficulty of sharing control is compounded by the nature of the environment in which clinicians practice, and the disenfranchised relationships and supports available to AIDS survivors.

Certain deaths are more difficult to resolve than others. Workers have reported that the death of a child to AIDS is most distressing. Clinicians are left with feelings similar to those of the parents. They continue to feel that somehow they should have been able to save and protect the child. Many young children die of AIDS within two years of diagnosis, and the factors governing length and quality of survival are not understood. The burden of care for adolescents diagnosed HIV-positive is just being recognized, and although not addressed here, has been an area of discomfort.

Regardless of the age of the person who has died of AIDS, professionals are called upon to give advice on some of the following issues: how to handle siblings and relatives; hospital procedures; routines with the funeral director; insurance and expenses. All of this occurs while the clinician is offering support in dealing with the emotional and physical pain survivors experience.

CLINICIANS WITH HIV/AIDS

Very difficult issues are raised when the clinician is HIV-positive or has developed symptoms of AIDS. The practitioner's reaction to a client's sexual style may be influenced by knowledge of her or his own HIV status and sexual life-style. This can both enhance and detract from the counseling relationship. On the one hand, it can serve to increase the capacity for empathy and the degree to which the clinician is perceived by the client as a potentially understanding helping person. On the other hand, the clinician can become overinvested and, due to emotional strain, be unable to continue the work. Self-absorption, a natural response to a personal crisis, makes it difficult to remain attuned to a client's problems and concerns.

Kaplan and Rothman (1986) state that while the concept of healthy denial may be useful to maintain day-to-day functioning, it can also distract both the professional and the client from experiencing the reality of illness, death, mourning and grief. Excessive despair and hopelessness may be an overwhelming burden for the clinician-survivor, and place the client in the role of the caretaker.

The need for consultation and/or therapy for practitioners who have HIV infection should be given a high priority. Several authors (Kaplan & Rothman 1986; Dewald 1982; Eissler 1973) have suggested that seriously and presumably terminally ill practitioners in private practice should refer their clients to another therapist while they still have time to go through a separation and termination phase with them.

A common feeling among social work clinicians is frustration over the high degree of ambiguity and the difficulty of identifying clear guidelines in helping survivors in a nonreceptive environment. AIDS and its ramifications confront professionals' own grief and unresolved feelings about death, homosexuality and drug use. If professionals are not vigilant, these unresolved feelings can interfere with the goal of providing safe, accepting environments for the expression of grief.

THE DEATH TOLL

Little is known empirically of the implications for professionals who are experiencing bereavement overload. This experience is not unlike the traumatic stress syndrome seen in those who survive floods, earthquakes, wars and the concentration camps during World War II. In recent years we have begun to address the psychosocial impact on the clinician of a caseload of persons with AIDS and their survivors. It is imperative to consider the multiple actual and anticipated losses of professionals working with this population. Those who care for people with AIDS and their families are affected by the stress of the ongoing health crisis. Watching young people die in the prime of life is a heavy emotional burden.

As a worker actively engages with people with AIDS, feelings of vulnerability parallel the potential threat of death that underlies the relationship process. Mourning reactions are prolific as clinicians grapple with serial losses. The effects of multiple losses compound a feeling of upheaval as practitioners learn that their system of beliefs and values has become ineffective. Loss and deprivation are inseparably bound together. Just as families have to cope with multiple deaths, so do professionals. Multiple deaths may result in common responses such as apathy, depression, guilt and loss of self-esteem.

Harper (1977) contends that the "maturing of the health professional" regarding their death-related coping strategies proceeds through five stages. The stages are intellectualization, emotional survival, depression, emotional arrival and deep compassion. Each of these stages produces corresponding psychological techniques and mechanisms—for example, pain, grief, mourning, self-actualization—that assist the professional in reducing anxiety about the client's death.

Confidence in one's ability to cope with the distress of others can be, and normally is, developed through a process of empathic attunement. Maintaining hope is a primary task for every professional, and it is one of the most difficult to sustain when working in the AIDS environment. Maintaining hope is a daily process; becoming aware of this requires reframing and redefining what feels hopeful. If hope is associated with more long-range goals, the professional will become frustrated. Active participation with one's family and friends, as well as finding meaning in day-to-day experiences, helps to maintain and strengthen feelings of hope for professionals who see clients, and in some cases friends, die of AIDS.

RESPONSES TO DEATH

Professionals committed to the care of people with AIDS and their survivors may well use occupationally devised strategies to deal with dying and multiple deaths. For instance, the coping strategies used by paramedics, as outlined by Palmer et al. (1984), are useful. They are (1) educational desensitization; (2) use of humor; (3) language alteration; (4) scientific fragmentation; (5) immersion in work; and (6) rationalization. Despite these coping strategies, paramedics still say that they sometimes are "angry as hell," "fedup," and "ready to chuck it all." These responses are similar to those of professionals working in the AIDS community.

Clinicians describe many coping strategies that help them deal with a client's death: attending the person's funeral, crying to exhaustion, requesting transfers to other units in the hospital and participating in group sessions to discuss their feelings. Many practitioners join an interagency support and resource group and feel reassured that they are not alone in their feelings. Knowing that others share your feelings somehow makes them less frightening and easier to deal with.

Some practitioners relate stories of nightmares and of being preoccupied with some clients, especially young children, under their care. They complain of "stressing out," "burning out," and "crashing." Some mention agency humor as a coping device. One theme resonates in all their comments: the conviction that in graduate school they were prepared for behavioral insights of clients, but not prepared for dealing with death and dying and the intensity of the emotions inherent in the grief process.

A way to become aware of the degree to which clinicians are responding to personal issues is for the professionals to strive to be more in touch with their internal experiences. Clinicians need to be sensitive to the physical sensations certain people trigger, the type of clients whom they find difficult to deal with, the fantasies they have about what others are thinking and the memories and feelings that certain situations arouse. Clinicians need to have self-awareness of their usual way of responding to particular kinds of people and relationships. This self-knowledge helps practitioners understand when they are responding to other people as external objects or when these responses are to internal objects and earlier relationships. From an object-relations perspective, it is clear that a person's experience of the world reflects her or his inner experience of self. Clinicians need the ability to differentiate external objects from internal objects and dialogues.

In order to cope with the emotional costs of repeated exposure to people who die, professionals gradually discover what they can do to alleviate distress, and how much of it is inevitable and insurmountable. Professionals vary widely in the extent to which they can do this. As long as they feel that their participation is worthwhile, they find themselves able to tolerate high levels of loss in others without disengaging.

Death always remains an enigma. Although professionals cannot solve the enigma, they can be provided with a better understanding of bereavement and be permitted to express feelings such as sadness or anger in a supportive and encouraging environment. Equally important is being aware of one's moment-to-moment experience. This awareness is a means by which practitioners grow and develop in their personal as well as professional lives, thus leading to even more productive and creative professional work.

EDUCATION AND SUPPORT OF STAFF MEMBERS

People with AIDS and their survivors require complex physiological, psychological and social interventions to meet their needs. Support and education of staff is crucial for maintaining the morale of social work professionals who daily serve on the front lines of AIDS work. In planning for staff training and development, administrators must take into consideration the extent to which clinicians possess the requisite knowledge and skills.

Medical, nursing, social work, psychology and counseling personnel have often had only minimal training in human sexuality. This deficit leaves them unfamiliar with sexual practices relevant to transmission and prevention, and may lead to fears of contagion. It is rare for training programs to teach students in the helping professions to deal with the behavior and the problems of gay persons, drug users or the sexually promiscuous. While African-American and Hispanic persons account for a disproportionately large number of AIDS cases, minority mental health and public health issues often receive only cursory attention in training programs or in post-graduate education (Kelly & St. Lawrence 1988).

Professional education and training must include information about people infected with HIV and AIDS and also deal with feelings about pain, illness, death and grief. Practitioners who understand their own histories of resolved or unresolved loss can be more effective in their bereavement work with clients. Understanding their style of coping and the processes they underwent before adequate resolution can be empowering. It can further help the clinician understand personal limitations with respect to the kinds of clients and the kinds of grief situations with which they can deal.

AIDS TRAINING

The acquisition of knowledge is a way of dispelling fear. Although much of this search for knowledge will be carried out by individuals, there remains a strong role for agency intervention.

Learning about AIDS, as with training on any other subject, succeeds or fails depending on how and whether the content touches the professional's experiences, values and beliefs, recalls their personal histories or challenges their assumptions. Providing facts alone is not a sufficient form of learning. Educational programs must take into account the varied cultural, religious and personal values affecting the clinician. For example, it is essential for clinicians to consider how they will respond when a client decides to bear a potentially infected child or to withhold information about AIDS diagnosis from a sexual partner.

Not only must practitioners be aware of their values, they must also understand how these values interfere in treatment. Enabling practitioners to understand their own reactions will help them to build counseling models to be used with the client and family members that focus on engagement and the giving of alternatives rather than on coercion.

Many staff members in today's work force, including those who serve PWAs, are young. Some may be single or just entering marriage or remarriage. In discussing high-risk behavior, we must be aware that some staff members may be participating in this type of sexual behavior. One also must not assume that it is only the youngest of the work force who may be sexually active outside a long-term monogamous relationship. Serial monogamy—a series of successive sexual involvements with one partner—may be practiced by many, regardless of age.

We posited earlier that few clinicians have been systematically trained to cope with issues of grief and bereavement. We have also indicated that the death of clients from AIDS affects clinicians in unique ways. Pursuant to these issues, we discussed in a previous publication (Dane & Miller 1990) both content and methodology specifically designed to prepare practitioners to cope with loss and death from AIDS.

In this approach, clinicians are systematically encouraged to examine their attitudes and reactions to death and dying in order to acquire general and specific knowledge about AIDS, and to develop clinical and counseling skills relevant to the psychosocial needs of those affected by the disease and their significant others. Handouts, focused questions, audio-visual materials, small group exercises, individual consultation and sensitive group discussions combine to enhance the clinician's self-awareness, increase potential for professional growth and maximize the ability to engage clients in facilitating grief work.

STAFF IN-SERVICE TRAINING

Education of staff at all levels is essential. A broad preventive approach should be used. Some agencies require attendance at a monthly AIDS meeting; writing articles about AIDS for the agency newspaper; informal discussions on recent medical, ethical and social issues; and the distribution of pamphlets or salient research, practice or policy journal articles.

Another educational approach is to bring in outside expert consultants to educate staff. Outside consultants can be identified through state and city health departments, regional business groups on health, the National Gay Task Force, regional hospitals, universities, the Centers for Disease Control and local AIDS-related organizations—for example, Gay Men's Health Crisis in New York City and the AIDS Foundation in San Francisco. A team of presenters is also recommended.

There are several advantages to employing outside consultants rather than using agency staff. First, they often have legitimacy in the eyes of the employees, since they are independent of the agency. Second, they have the latest information and expertise, which few health professionals would have.

Credibility is critically important, and the educator must be confident about the material. Third, consultants have experience in handling the kinds of questions and fears that arise in such situations, and they usually effectively reduce anxiety and calmly provide accurate information. Also, professionals may prefer to speak with outside consultants because outsiders are more objective and less potentially threatening. It may be easier to be open with someone not otherwise involved in judging the professional. Questions may be more easily expressed.

Hepworth, Schmidt and Sinapi (1986) developed an educational program for health care professionals that includes three components: a factual presentation about epidemiology and transmission of HIV, a videotaped personal account from a person with AIDS, and a small group discussion in which the personal implications of the facts are considered. The latter is stimulated by a discussion questionnaire containing controversial statements about AIDS. An important goal is to help professionals recognize that personal values affect decisions regarding health care and policy.

Small study groups, meeting on a weekly basis to discuss the challenges, dilemmas and difficulties of the work, are recommended. The group may focus on case presentations. Clipping daily newspaper articles about AIDS can help professional staff members keep in touch with recent and ever-changing developments. Because research developments occur quickly, information becomes out-of-date and insufficient very rapidly. When the professional is insufficiently concerned, judgmental or fails to understand the life-style of the client, little effective social and psychological intervention can be accomplished.

Some staff groups or individual members may have limited knowledge of issues of loss, death and bereavement. This can affect both their sense of competence and their work with clients. Agency administrators can provide consultation or appropriate literature addressing specific themes. Ideally, the administrator can arrange for systematic development of AIDS education for the entire staff. The objective and techniques of psychoeducation (Miller 1986), currently used with clients and nonprofessional caregivers, can be adapted for such use. Over a six-week period, the following themes can be addressed, with emphasis on their implications for practice with grievers: (1) loss—meaning and needs of the bereaved; (2) consequences of unresolved grief; (3) role of the professional caregiver for the bereaved; (4) interventive strategies; (5) impact on the professional; and (6) care and support of the clinician.

The composition of the small groups, designed to discuss attitudes, fears and worries about AIDS as well as knowledge and interventive skills, is critical to the success of the endeavor. Group composition has implications for the freedom with which individuals express their concerns, share their successes and failures or ask for information and help in a mutual aid context. One administrator reports that the bonding of gay men in one group of professionals tacitly communicated the notion that female staff members could not understand what it was like to live with AIDS or to be left behind when your lover dies. Group leaders need to handle the dynamics and splits in small groups and to be attentive to the ongoing process.

As the magnitude of the AIDS crisis expands, professionals who have never been involved with AIDS-affected persons and their bereaved survivors will develop interests in the area or will find themselves in the position of counseling this population. To understand extremely complex issues in working with these groups, comprehensive training for professionals should include experiential, medical, psychosocial and legal issues.

The format for educational sessions can vary: one-on-one supervision or counseling, small group meetings, seminars, workshops or large-scale question-and-answer sessions are among the possibilities. Ideally, education should be targeted to all employees, but occasionally educational efforts are limited to those who are actually involved in working with people with AIDS or their survivors. A staff person or a volunteer committee in a large agency can be assigned the task of AIDS-related education, and can poll the staff regarding their interests.

ASSESSING AND PREVENTING BURNOUT

The pervasiveness of publications on burnout would suggest that it occurs in virtually every job setting. Work stresses adversely affecting health care practitioners have received a great deal of attention. Burnout among health professionals has been documented for the past fifteen years (Cherniss 1980; Freudenberger 1982; Harrison 1980; Jayaratne & Chess 1984; Maslach 1976, 1981; Pines & Kafry 1978), but little has been documented in the area of professionals working with persons with AIDS and their survivors.

Burnout is sometimes loosely defined. In characterizing a worker as burned out, we are not pointing to the transient, temporary feelings that every worker experiences when a case has blown up. The term is validly applicable only to a persistent, chronic condition, which results from a cumulative, prolonged and undissipated buildup of stress.

Maslach (1981) guides our discussion with her definition. She defines burnout as "a syndrome of emotional exhaustion, depersonalization, and reduced personal accomplishment that [occurs in response to]... the chronic emotional strain of dealing extensively with other human beings, particularly when they are troubled or having problems." (1).

This description of burnout is certainly consistent with what is experienced by professionals in AIDS work, where emotional overload and stress-inducing work with illness, loss and death proliferate. In recent years, there has been an increasing awareness of the need to develop specific techniques for helping mental health professionals alleviate the complex problems of burnout, especially when working with bereaved families after a great deal of work has been undertaken prior to the person's death.

Most professionals have a mental image of a person who suffers from burnout, but they seldom recognize the slow, insidious change from an energetic, enthusiastic person to one who is exhausted and apathetic. Colleagues too are affected by a person suffering from burnout, and it is imperative to recognize and prevent the process. The process of burnout is a gradual one.

Patrick (1984) outlines the characteristics that describe persons who burn out. It is obvious that these are positive qualities to which most practitioners aspire, and which administrators seek in prospective employees. The operative concept is that these are qualities that should be present in moderation, and counterbalanced by non-work sources of personal and professional self-fulfillment. The characteristics include the following:

- Enthusiasm
- Independence
- Compassion
- Intensity
- Motivation
- Quality orientation
- Energetic manner
- Self-starting ability
- Achievement orientation
- Ambition
- High expectations
- Self-sufficiency
- Sensitivity
- Clear goals (27)

Additional characteristics might include idealism, impatience or low frustration tolerance. These powerful positive characteristics, all essential in AIDS work, can make a professional susceptible to burnout.

Although there is some controversy regarding the validity of the burnout concept, few experts deny the reality of the end-product loss of highly educated and skilled professionals to the field of AIDS practice. Creative thinking, analysis and well-planned interventions designed to ameliorate or eliminate professional burnout are sorely needed. While we are working on long-term solutions to the problems created by burnout, strategies to promote retention of professionals in AIDS work address the preventive, interventive and management aspects of the burnout issue.

PROACTIVE PLANNING

A proactive stance is recommended in thinking about and planning ahead for working with persons with AIDS and their survivors. Learning about AIDS, bereavement and death, exploring options for handling problems, getting the facts on coverage, traditional and experimental drugs, support groups and other community resources, as well as confronting the ethical issues encountered in the work, are ways to avoid crises. Finding oneself prepared tends to encourage and promote competency, and is therefore self-empowering. Clinicians must be aware that some factors are beyond immediate agency control, such as deficient community resources, staff or funding cutbacks, heavy client resistance and a high death toll.

INDIVIDUAL ASSESSMENT

Determining the degree to which a practitioner is experiencing burnout is not an easy task. Only the person experiencing it is aware of her/his current feelings as compared with feelings experienced in the past. Stress can be escalated as a result of working with chronically ill, dying people and their survivors. Some monitoring of staff behaviors to indicate burnout should be in effect. The following list of behaviors, outlined by Harris (1984), can be used as a guideline:

- *Change in communication with others*: Interchanges between the professional and colleagues are heated and curt. Also, the professional seems to be speaking less to others, often only when spoken to first.
- *Isolation*: The professional does not participate with the work group as he or she had done previously.
- *Increased work errors*: The quality of work has decreased.
- *Increased use of sick time*: The professional is experiencing either stress-related illness, such as gastrointestinal disturbances, headaches and colds, or increased accidents.
- *Decrease in risk-taking behaviors*: The professional seems unable to make decisions and has become less flexible.
- *Increased use of overtime in small increments*: The previously efficient worker begins to need more time to accomplish the same amount of work.
- *Chronic tardiness*: The professional may be experiencing increasing difficulty in getting out of bed to get to work on time because of a dislike of work or increasing feelings of burnout.

All of these behaviors, singly or collectively, can be the result of difficulties other than burnout. It is essential for the supervisor to address these behaviors and find a method to alleviate the distress in a positive and supportive manner.

ORGANIZATIONAL ASSESSMENT

In assessing burnout one must also include an organizational assessment to refrain from blaming the professional and to allow for framing the difficulty in a holistic manner. An effective way of assessing organizational burnout is to examine the cultural norms and values of the agency and consider the following variables (Harris 1984, 35-38):.

- *Bureaucratization*: How many layers of administration are present? Is the organizational chart clear to all? Do the employees know the accountability relationships of their immediate supervisor?

- *Communication*: How do the frontline workers rate the effectiveness of communication? How many methods of communication are available to frontline workers?

- *Level of decision-making*: How much influence do frontline workers have on decisions-made about their work? Is decision-making participatory? Do unit problems get solved at the unit or at a higher level of administration?

- *Role models*: Is there congruence between the verbal and nonverbal behavior of the role model? Are informal role models the same as the organizational role models?

- *Job expectations*: Are all professionals, including supervisor and staff, clear about what is expected of them in their specific job roles? Do they feel comfortable clarifying confusion about expectations?

- *Physical environment*: Is there a staff lounge available? Do supervisors have adequate office space to carry out confidential conversations and shut out extraneous noise?

- *Psychological environment*: Are creative ideas welcomed? Are there sufficient resources available for job completion? Is there room for movement among professionals within the system? Is employee health and well-being important to the agency?

The following areas of behavior might reveal trends that could help determine which groups of workers might be having more trouble than others: sick time, vacation time, incident reports, on-the-job accidents, overtime, worker transfer to another unit and worker resignation.

These are some of the behaviors cited by Harris (1984) that should be examined in attempting to assess the organization for potential burnout hazards or causes of existing burnout. These behaviors can be applied to professionals working with people with AIDS and their bereaved survivors.

By encouraging and structuring support for its staff, an institution demonstrates that it is aware of and concerned about the stress inherent in working with an AIDS population. The agency's responsibility to help its clients includes an acknowledgment of the stressful effects of multiple deaths and ongoing mourning of agency staff, and of the impact management and organizational practices can have on staff functioning in these stressful settings.

GUIDELINES FOR DEALING WITH STRESS

Much of the literature emphasizes self-directed approaches as ways to prevent burnout. Ratliff (1988) suggests personal therapy, setting boundaries to allow for personal time, realistic goal-setting, and the development of health support systems. Interventions that focus largely on the adaptation of individuals and cosmetic changes to the system have been suggested by a number of writers (Cherniss 1980). McNeeley (1988) points to the failure of individual solutions for the management of stress and of efforts to restructure organizations in response to burnout. He outlines such options as "leisure sharing," whereby workers may exchange a percentage of their salaries for extended time off, job sharing, flexible benefit packages and the use of quality circles for participatory problem-solving.

To reduce burnout and stress for those professionals who work with PWAs and their survivors, a holistic view is required. The integration of individual and institutional strategies to work toward establishing environments of mutual support must begin with a commitment to empowerment.

The social environment is not just a major source of stress, it also provides vital resources that the professional as a survivor can and must draw upon in order to endure and flourish. That people gain sustenance and support from social relationships has been known intuitively for a long time.

Schaefer, Coyne & Lazarus (1982) distinguish three functions of social support. These are emotional support (including attachment, reassurance and being able to rely on and confide in a person), which contributes to the feeling that one is loved or cared about; tangible support (involving direct aid such as loans or gifts, and services such as taking care of someone who is ill, doing a job or chore, etc.); and informational support (providing information or advice, and giving feedback about how a person is doing). Cassel (1976) suggests that feedback helps the person maintain social identity and a sense of integration in society. Tangible support, when proffered freely and voluntarily, may signal that the other person cares and that the recipient is valued, and in this way it can overlap with emotional support.

Worden (1982) suggests three guidelines in working with the bereaved, which can be applied to AIDS work. The first is to know your own limitations in terms of the number of clients with whom you can work intimately and be attached to at any given time. To the extent that there is an attachment, there is going to be a loss that the practitioner will need to grieve. Second, when a person dies it is important to go through a period of active grieving, to experience the sadness and other feelings after someone dies, and not to feel guilty for not grieving to the same degree for each person. Third, the clinician should know how to reach out for help and know how to identify personal sources of support. Many times professionals find it easier to help others than to negotiate for their own need to be helped with their grief.

Professionals as survivors need emotional support, training, supervision and the opportunity to explore their styles of coping. When these elements are available, practitioners will function better and have a higher level of job satisfaction.

FUTURE HOPES AND EXPECTATIONS

The era when AIDS, and concentrated efforts to cope with its implications, were in the forefront of societal concern is ending. This has resurged with the disclosures of Arthur Ashe and Magic Johnson. There continues howeve to be a decrease in resources available to programs, lack of attention paid by the media and the decrease of public outrage related to this epidemic. Yet the number of practitioners interested in working with PWAs and their survivors continues to grow. One can assume that this growth will continue for the immediate future, balancing the numbers of experienced practitioners who leave after expending their emotional and physical energy. Every effort must be made to maintain and build on the emotional and physical investment of the practitioner new to AIDS work and to shore up the reserves of those who have worked in this area of practice for many years. Creating support groups in the workplace, in which a practitioner can feel safe to express a range of feelings and to grieve, is vital. This need is exacerbated as the practitioner experiences multiple deaths.

We can anticipate continued public ambivalence about AIDS and about anyone associated with the disease. Practitioners, as a result, will need to have their thoughts and actions confirmed by others who are significant to them, such as supervisors and administrators. Political figures and funding sources can demonstrate support by sustaining and increasing funding for current and needed programs for bereaved survivors.

Given the continued academic and professional investment in AIDS, indicated by the number of participants attending national and international conferences and the vast number of books and articles on the topic, it is inevitable that the breadth of knowledge and information will continue to increase. The need to assist practitioners in keeping abreast of this expanse of information has been mentioned above. The hope is that practitioners will see themselves as contributing to this enterprise. Those who intervene on the front line have a unique perspective on the problems encountered by PWAs and their bereaved survivors. Sharing this perspective beyond the immediate confines of their programs serves as an outlet for their motivations and enthusiasm for helping those in grief. It can further be useful to those contemplating working with the bereaved.

Forecasters do not anticipate the eradication of the AIDS disease in this century, or in the first decades of the twenty-first century. New paradigms for professional cooperation are emerging to eradicate the formidable emotional and social stressors that people with AIDS and their survivors experience. Tremendous personal and professional accomplishments are possible if one not only becomes involved in AIDS work directly but engages in political activities to stem the epidemic.

The essential hope is that practitioners, politicians and the general public muster the commitment and energy and generate the resources to answer the question posed so eloquently by Tiblier, Walker and Roland (1989): How best can our society provide compassionate and effective medical and mental health care, cover the enormous financial and emotional cost of AIDS, help families find the internal resources necessary to grow through the grief of infection, illness and death, and create a safer and more humane environment for us all? (p.122-23).

Bibliography

Adelman, M. (1989). Social support and AIDS. *AIDS & Public Policy Journal*, *4*, 31-39.

Aguilar, I., & Wood, V. N. (1976). Aspects of death, grief and mourning in the treatment of Spanish-speaking mental patients. *Social Work*, *21*, 49-54.

Airhihenbuwa, C. (1989). Perspectives on AIDS in Africa: Strategies for prevention & control. *AIDS: Education and Prevention: An Interdisciplinary Journal*, *1*, 57-69.

Albert, E. (1986). Illness & deviance: The response of the press to AIDS. In D. A. Feldman & T. M. Johnson (Eds.), *The social dimension of AIDS* (163-178). NY: Praeger.

Albrecht, T. L., & Adelman, M. B. (1987). Communicating social support: A theoretical perspective. In T. L. Albrecht & M. B. Adelman (Eds.), *Communicating social support* (18-39). Newbury Park, CA: Sage Publications.

Aldrich, C. K. (1974). Some dynamics of anticipatory grief. In B. Schoenberg, A. Carr, A. Kutscher, D. Peretz & I. Goldberg (Eds.), *Anticipatory grief* (3-47). NY: Columbia University Press.

Altman, D. (1986). *AIDS in the mind of America*. NY: Anchor Press/Doubleday.

Altman, L. (1991). Report on international AIDS meeting. *New York Times*, July, 18, A27.

Anderson, G. (1990). *Courage to cure: Responding to the crisis of children with AIDS*. Washington, D.C.: Child Welfare League of America.

Bacon, L. (1987). Lessons of AIDS: Racism, homophobia, the real epidemic. *Listen Real Loud*, *8*, 5-6.

Balk, D. (1983). Effects of sibling death on teenagers. *Journal of School Health*, *27*, 14-18.

Ball, J. (1977). Widows' grief: The impact of age & mode of death. *Omega*, *7*, 303-323.

Bandura, A. (1977). Self-efficacy: Toward a unifying theory of behavioral change. *Psychological Review*, *84*, 191-215.

———. (1982). Self-efficacy mechanisms in human agency. *American Psychologist*, *37*, 122-147.

Barrett, C. J. (1978). Effectiveness of widows' groups in facilitating change. *Journal of Consulting & Clinical Psychology*, *46*, 20-31.

Barrows, P. A., & Halgin, R. P. (1988). Current issues in psychotherapy with gay men: Impact of the AIDS phenomenon. *Professional Psychology: Research and Practice*, *19*, 395-402.

Batchelor, W. F. (1984). AIDS. *American Psychologist*, *39*, 1277-1278.

Bayer, R. (1989). AIDS, privacy & responsibility. *Daedalus, Living with AIDS Summer Part II, Journal of the American Academy of Arts and Sciences*, 79-100.

Bell, A. P., & Weinberg, M. S. (1978). *Homosexualities: A study of diversity among men and women*, NY: Simon and Schuster. Bettelheim, B. (1979). *Surviving and other essays*. NY: Alfred A. Knopf.

Bettelheim, B. (1979). *Surviving and other essays*. NY: Alfred A. Knopf.

Black, D. (1985). *The plague years: A chronicle of AIDS, the epidemic of our times*, NY: Simon and Schuster.

Bloom, J. R. (1982). Social support systems and cancer: A conceptual view. In J. Cohen, J. W. Cullen & L. R. Martin (Eds.), *Psychosocial aspects of cancer* (129-149). NY: Raven Press.

Blumberg, B., Flaherty, M. & Lewis, J. (Eds.). (1980). *Coping with cancer: A resource for the health professional*. Bethesda, MD: National Cancer Institute.

Blumfield, M., Smith, P., Milazzio, J., Seropian, S. & Wormser, G. (1987). Survey of attitudes of nurses working with AIDS patients. *General Hospital Psychiatry*, *9*, 58-63.

Bolin, R. C. (1982). *Long-term family recovery from disaster*, University of Colorado, Institute of Behavioral Science. Program on environment and behavior, Monograph no. 36.

Bonkowski, S., Bequette, S. & Boomhower, S. (1984). A group designed to help children adjust to parental divorce. *Social Casework*, *65*, 131-137.

Boss, P. (1988). *Family stress management*, Newbury Park, CA: Sage Publications.

Bowen, M. (1978). *Family therapy in clinical practice*. NY: Jacob Aronson.

———. (1987). Family reaction to death. In P. Guerin (Ed.), *Family therapy* (335-348). NY: Gardner Press.

Bowen, O. (1987). Preface in O. R. Bowen (Ed.), *AIDS: Information/education plan to prevent and control AIDS in the United States* (1-11). Washington, D.C.: U.S. Department of Health & Human Services, Public Health Service.

Bowlby, J. (1951). *Maternal care and mental health*. World Health Organization Monograph no. 2.

———. (1960). Separation anxiety. *International Journal of Psychoanalysis*, *41*, 89-113.

———. (1961). Childhood mourning and its implications for psychiatry. *American Journal of Psychiatry*, *118*, 481-498.

———. (1969). *Attachment and loss*, Vol. 1 London: Hogarth; NY: Basic Books.

———. (1973). *Attachment and loss*, Vol. 2. *Separation anxiety and anger*, NY: Basic Books.

———. (1977). The making and breaking of affectional bonds. *British Journal of Psychiatry*, *130*, 201-210.

———. (1980a). *Attachment and loss*, Vol. 3. *Loss: Sadness and depression*. NY: Basic Books.

————. (1980b). *Loss: Sadness and depression*. London: Hogarth, NY: Basic Books.

————. (1980c). *Separation: Anxiety and anger*, Vol. 3. London: Hogarth; NY: Basic Books.

Boyd-Franklin, N. (1989). *Black families in therapy: A multisystems approach*. NY: Guilford Press.

Brown, C. (1965). *Manchild in the promised land*. NY: Signet Books.

Brown, G. W., & Harris, T. (1978). *Social origins of depression*. NY: Free Press.

Brown, L. (1989). Lesbians, gay men and their families: Common clinical issues. *Journal of Gay and Lesbian Psychotherapy, 1*, 65-77.

Bugen, L. A. (1977). Human grief: A model for prediction and intervention. *American Journal of Orthopsychiatry, 47*, 196-205.

Caplan, G. (1961). *Prevention of mental disorders in children: Initial Exploration*. NY: Basic Books.

Caplan, G., & Killilea, M. (Eds.). (1976). *Support systems and mutual help*. NY: Grune and Stratton.

Caputo, L. (1985). Dual diagnosis: AIDS and addiction. *Social Work, 30*, 361-364.

Carey, J. S. (1988). Routine preoperational screening for HIV. *Journal of the American Medical Association, 260*, 179.

Carter, B., & McGoldrick, M. (Eds.) (1989). *The changing family life cycle: A framework for family therapy*. 2nd ed. Boston: Allyn & Bacon.

Cassel, J. (1976). The contribution of the social environment to past resistance. *American Journal of Epidemiology, 104*, 107-123.

Centers for Disease Control. (1986). *Acquired immunodeficiency syndrome (AIDS) weekly surveillance report: United States AIDS program*. Atlanta, GA.

————. (1988). CDC surveillance summaries. *Morbidity and Mortality Weekly Report, 37*, 4-7.

————. (1990a). HIV prevalence estimates and AIDS case projections for the United States: Report based upon a workshop. *Morbidity and Mortality Weekly Report, 39*, 1-13.

————. (1990b). Update: Acquired immunodeficiency syndrome—United States, 1989. *Morbidity and Mortality Weekly Report, 39*, 81-86.

Cherniss, C. (1980). *Staff burnout: Job stress in the human services*. Beverly Hills, CA: Sage Publications.

Chestang, L. (1976). Environmental influences on social functioning: The black experience. In P. Cafferty & L. Chestang (Eds.), *The diverse society: Implications for social policy* (59-74). NY: Association Press.

Chodoff, P. (1985). Psychiatric aspects of the Nazi persecutions. In S. Ariete (Ed.), *American Handbook of Psychiatry*. NY: Basic Books.

Christ, G. H., & Wiener, L. S. (1985). Psychosocial issues in AIDS. In V. T. De Vita, Jr., S. Hellman & S. Rosenberg (Eds.), *AIDS etiology diagnosis treatment and prevention* (275-297). Philadelphia, PA: J. B. Lippincott.

Christakis, N. (1989). Responding to a pandemic: International interests in AIDS control. *Daedalus, I, Journal of the American Academy of Arts and Sciences*, 113-134.

Clark, G. M. (Ed.). (1986). *Legal issues in transfusion medicine*. Arlington, VA: American Association of Blood Banks.

Clark, H., Westley, L. & Washburn, P. (1988). Testing for human immunodeficiency virus in substance abuse treatment. *Journal of Psychoactive Drugs, 20*, 203-211.

Cleveland, P. H., Walters, L. H., Skeen, P. & Robinson, B. E. (1988). If your child had AIDS . . . : Responses of parents with homosexual children. *Family Relations, 37,* 150-153.

Clever, L. H., & Omann, G. S. (1988). Hazards for health care workers. *Annual Review of Public Health, 9,* 273-303.

Coates, D., Renzaglia, G. J. & Embree, M. C. (1983). When helping backfires: Help and helplessness. In J. D. Fisher, A. Nadler & B. De Paulo (Eds.), *New directions in helping: Recipient reactions to aid.* Vol. 1. NY: Academic Press.

Coates, T. J., Stall, R., Mandell, J. S., Baccellari, A., Sorensen, J. L., Morales, E., Morin, S., Wiley, J. & McKusky, L. (1987). AIDS: A psychosocial research agenda. *Annals of Behavioral Medicine, 9,* 21-28.

Coates, T. J., Temoshok, L. & Mandel, J. (1984). Psychosocial research is essential to understanding and treating AIDS. *American Psychologist, 39,* 1309-1304.

Cohen, M. M., & Willisch, D. K. (1978). Living in limbo: Psychological intervention in families with a cancer patient. *American Journal of Psychotherapy, 32,* 561-571.

Cohen, P., Dizenhuz, I. M. & Winget, C. (1977). Family adaptation to terminal illness and death of a parent. *Social Casework, 58,* 223-228.

Cohen, R. E., & Ahearn, F. C. (1980). *Handbook for mental health care victims.* Baltimore, MD: Johns Hopkins University Press.

Cohen, S. & Willis, J. A. (1985). Stress, social support and the buffering hypotheses. *Psychological Bulletin,* 98, 310-357.

Corless, I. B., & Pittman-Lindeman, M. (Eds.). (1988). *AIDS: Principles, practice and politics.* NY: Hemisphere Publ. Corp.

Cowan, M. E., & Murphy, S. A. (1985). Identification of past disaster bereavement risk predictions. *Nursing Research, 34,* 71-75.

Curran, J. W., & Jaffe, L. (1985). The epidemiology and prevention of the acquired immuno-deficiency syndrome. *American International Medicine, 103,* 657-662.

Curran, J. W., Morgan, W. M., Hardy, A. M., Jaffe, H., Darrow, W. & Dowale, W. (1985). The epidemiology of AIDS: Current status and future prospects. *Science, 229,* 1352-1357.

Dalton, H. (1989). AIDS in Blackface in living with AIDS. *Daedalus, Part II, Living with Aids. Journal of the American Academy of Arts & Sciences,* 1205-1228.

Dane, B. O. (1989). New beginnings for AIDS patients. *Social Casework: The Journal of Contemporary Social Work, 70,* 305-309.

―――. (1990). Death of a child. In A. Gitterman (Ed.), *Handbook of social work practice with vulnerable populations* (112-132). NY: Columbia University Press.

Dane, B., & Miller, S. O. (1990). AIDS and dying: The teaching challenge. *Journal of Teaching in Social Work, 4,* 85-100.

Danieli, Y. (1985). The treatment and prevention of long-term effects and intergenerational transmission of victimization: A lesson from holocaust survivors and their children. In C. Figley (Ed.), *Trauma and its wake* (295-313). NY: Brenner/Mazel.

Davidowitz, M., & Myreck, R. (1984). Responding to the bereaved: An analysis of "helping" statements. *Death Education, 8,* 5-7.

Dersheimer, R. A. (1990). *Counseling the bereaved.* NY: Pergamon Press.

Dewald, P. A. (1982). Serious illness in the analyst: Transference, countertransference and reality response. *Journal of the American Psychoanalytic Association, 30,* 347-363.

Dilley, J. W., Pies, C. & Helquist, M. (1989). *Face to face: A guide to AIDS counselling,* Berkeley, CA: Celestial Arts.

Doka, K. J. (1987). Silent sorrow: Grief and the loss of significant others. *Death Studies, 11,* 455-469.

———. (1989). *Disenfranchised grief: Recognizing hidden sorrow.* Lexington, MA: Lexington Books.

Douglas, C. J., Kalman, C. M. & Kalman, T. P. (1985). Homophobia among physicians and nurses: An empirical study. *Hospital and Community Psychiatry, 36,* 1309-1311.

Drucker, E. (1991). AIDS and addiction in New York City. *American Journal of Drug and Alcohol Abuse, 12,* 165-181.

Dumont, R., & Foss, D. (1972). *The American view of death.* Cambridge, MA: Schenkmore Publishing.

Dunkel, J., & Hatfield, S. (1986). Countertransference issues in working with persons with AIDS. *Social Work, 31,* 114-117.

Dupree, J. D., & Margo, C. (1988). Homophobia, AIDS and the health care professional. *Focus, 3,* 1-2.

Eissler, K. R. (1973). On the possible effects of aging on the practice of psychoanalysis. *Journal of the Philadelphia Association for Psychoanalysis, 3,* 138-152.

Eliot, G. (1972). *The twentieth-century book of the dead.* London: Allen Lane.

Engel, G. L. (1961). Is grief a disease? A challenge for medical research. *Psychosomatic Medicine, 23,* 18-22.

———. (1964). Grief & grieving. *American Journal of Nursing, 64,* 93-98.

Epstein, Y., & Bordin, C. (1985). Could this happen? A game for children of divorce. *Psychotherapy, 22,* 770-773.

Erikson, E. H. (1950). *Childhood and society.* NY: W. W. Norton.

Eth, S., & Pynoos, R. (1985). *Post-traumatic stress disorder in children.* Washington, D.C.: American Psychiatric Press.

Falicov, C. J. (1982). Mexican families. In M. McGoldrick, J. K. Pearce & J. Giordano (Eds.), *Ethnicity and family therapy* (371). NY: Guilford Press.

Figley, C. (Ed.). (1985). *Trauma and its wake.* NY: Brenner/Mazel.

———. (1988). Victimization, trauma and traumatic stress. *The Counselling Psychologist, 16,* 635-641.

Fischer, E. J. (1986). How to combat the AIDS epidemic. *Michigan Medicine, 85,* March, 93-102.

Fischer, J. (1988). Possible effects of reference group-based social influence on AIDS-risk behavior and AIDS prevention. *American Psychologist, 43,* 914-920.

Flaskerud, J. H. (Ed.). (1987). Special Issue: AIDS—The psychosocial dimension. *Journal of Psychosocial Nursing, 25,* 9-16.

Flesch, (1976). The clergy on the firing line. In. V. R. Pine, A. Kutscher, D. Peretz, R. Slater, R. DeBellis, R. Volk & D. Cherico (Eds.), *Acute grief and the funeral,* Springfield, IL: Charles Thomas.

Folkman, S. (1984). *Stress, appraisal and coping.* NY: Springer Publishing.

Folta, J. R., & Deck, E. S. (1974). *Grief, the funeral, and the friend.* Paper presented at the Foundation of Thanatology. New York.

Fossum, M. A., & Mason, M. J. (1986). *Facing shame.* NY: W. W. Norton.

Foster, Z. (1988). The treatment of people with AIDS: Psychosocial considerations. In I. B. Corless & M. Puttman Lindeman (Eds.), *AIDS: Principles, practice and politics*. NY: Hemisphere Publishing.

Friedland, G. (1989). Clinical care in the AIDS epidemic. *Daedalus, Living with AIDS*, Part I, Spring, *Journal of the American Academy of Arts and Sciences*, *118*, 59-84.

Freidland, G., & Klein, S. (1987). Recommendations for prevention of HIV transmission in health care settings. *Morbidity and Mortality, Weekly Report, 3625*, 3-18.

Freud, A. (1957). Mourning and melancholia. In J. Richman (Ed.), *A general selection from the works of Sigmund Freud* (86-101). NY: Doubleday.

———. (1960). Discussion of Dr. Bowlby's Paper. *Psychoanalytic Study of the Child*, *15*, 53.

———. (1963). Beyond the pleasure principle. NY: Bantam Books.

Freud, S. (1894). *The neuro-psychoses of defense*, 3. Standard Edition. London: Hogarth.

———. (1917). *Mourning and melancholia*, 14. Standard Edition, London: Hogarth.

Freudenberger, H. with G. Richelieu (1982). *Burnout: The high cost of high achievement*. Garden City, NY: Anchor Press.

Freudenberger, W., Lee, J. & Silver, D. (1989). How Black and Latino community organizations respond to the AIDS epidemic: A case study in one New York City neighborhood. *AIDS Education and Prevention*, *1*, 12-21.

Fudin, C., & Devore, W. (1981). The unidentified bereaved. In O. S. Margolis, H. C. Raether, A. H. Kutscher, J. B. Powers, I. B. Seeland, R. DeBellis & D. J. Cherico (Eds.), *Acute grief: Counselling the bereaved* (133-142). NY: Columbia University Press.

Fulmer, R. (1989). Lower-income and professional families: A comparison of structure and life cycle process. In B. Carter & M. McGoldrick (Eds.), *The changing family life cycle: A framework for family therapy* (545-578). Boston: Allyn and Bacon.

Fulton, R. (1987). The many faces of grief. *Death Studies*, *11*, 243-256.

Fulton, R., & Owen, G. (1988). AIDS: seventh rank absolute in AIDS. In I. B. Corless, B. Pittman Lindeman (Eds.), *AIDS Principles, practices and politics* (237-249). Washington, D.C.: Hemisphere Publishing.

Furman, E. (1974). *A child's parent dies: Studies in childhood bereavement*. New Haven, CT: Yale University Press.

Gagnon, J. H. (1983). Reviews of the literature. *American Journal of Orthopsychiatry*, *53*, 560-568.

———. (1989). Disease and desire. *Daedalus, Living with AIDS: Part II. Journal of the American Academy of Arts and Sciences*, 47-78.

Gagnon, J. H., & Greenblatt, C. S. (1977). Health care planning and education via gaming—Simulation's a two-stage experiment. *Health Education Monographs Supplement*.

Garcia-Preto, N. (1982). Puerto Rican families. In M. McGoldrick, J. K. Pearce & J. Giordano (Eds.), *Ethnicity and family therapy* (164-186). NY: Guilford Press.

Gardner, R. (1983). *Children: Reactions to parental death*. In J. Schowalter, P. Patterson, M. Tallmer, A. Kutscher, S. Gullo & D. Peretz (Eds.), *The Child and Death* (104-124). NY: Columbia University Press.

Garfield, C. (1979). A child dies. In C. A. Garfield (Ed.), *Stress and survival* (314-317). St. Louis, MO: C. V. Mosby.

Garrett, J. E. (1988). The AIDS patient: Helping him and his parents cope. *Nursing*, *18*, 50-53.

Gauthier, J., & Marshall, W. L. (1977). Grief: A cognitive behavioural analysis. *Cognitive Therapy and Research*, *1*, 39-44.

Geis, S. B., Fuller, R. L. & Rush, J. (1986). Lovers of AIDS victims: Psychosocial stresses and counseling needs. *Death Studies*, *10*, 43-53.

Gerbert, B. (1987). AIDS and infection control in dental practice: Dentists' knowledge, attitudes and behaviors. *Journal of the American Dental Association*, *114*, 311-314.

Gerbert, B., Badner, V. & Maguire, B. (1988). AIDS and dental practice. *Journal of Public Health Denistry*, *48*, 68-73.

Getzel, G. (1990). AIDS. In A. Gitterman (Ed.), *Handbook of social work practice with vulnerable populations* (35-64). NY: Columbia University Press.

Gilbert, J. (1988). Coming to terms. *Family Therapy Networker*, *12*, 42-43.

Glaser, B., & Strauss, A. (1967). *The discovery of grounded theory; strategies for qualitative research*. Chicago: Aldine Publishing.

Glick, I., Weiss, R. & Parkes, M. (1974). *The first year of bereavement*. NY: John Wiley & Sons.

Glick, I. O., Weiss, R. & Parkes, C. M., (1974). *The first year of bereavement*. NY: John Wiley & Sons.

Goffman, E. (1963). *Stigma: Notes on the management of spoiled identity*. Englewood Cliffs, NJ: Prentice-Hall.

Gonda, M. (1986). The natural history of AIDS. *Natural History*, *95*, 78-81.

Gonsiorek, J. C. (1982). An introduction to mental health issues and homosexuality. *American Behavioral Scientist*, *25*, 367-384.

Gordon, D. (1978). *Therapeutic Metaphors: Helping others through the looking glass*. Cupertino, CA: Meta Publications.

Gorer, G. (1965). *Death, grief and mourning*. NY: Doubleday.

Gottlieb, B. H. (1978). The development and application of a classification scheme of informal helping behaviors. *Canadian Journal of Science*, *10*, 105-115.

Greenberg, L. (1975). Therapeutic grief work with children. *Social Casework*, *56*, 396-403.

Greif, G. L., & Porembski, E. (1988). AIDS and significant others: Findings from a preliminary exploration of needs. *Health and Social Work*, *13*, 259-265.

Guinan, M. E., & Hardy, A. (1987). Epidemiology of AIDS in women in the United States: 1981-1986. *Journal of the American Medical Association*, *257*, 2039-2042.

Haan, N. (1977). *Coping and defending: Processes of self-environment organization*. NY: Academic Press.

Hanley, L., & Hackenbruck P. (1989). Psychotherapy and the "coming out" process. *Journal of Gay and Lesbian Psychotherapy*, *1*, 21-39.

Hare-Mustin, R. (1979). Family therapy following the death of a child. *Journal of Marital and Family Therapy*, *5*, 51-59.

Harper, B. (1977). *Death: The coping mechanism of the health professional*. Greenville, South Carolina: Southeastern University Press.

Harris, P. (1984). Assessing burnout: The organizational and individual perspective. *Family and Community Health*, *2*, 32-43.

Harrison, W. (1980). Role strain and burnout in child protective service workers. *Social Service Review*, *54*, 31-44.

Hartsough, P. M. (1985). Measurement of the psychological effects of disaster. In J. Laurie & S. A. Murphy (Eds.), *Perspectives on disaster recovery* (22-60). East Norwalk, CT: Appleton-Century Crofts.

Hepworth, J., Schmidt, P. & Sinapi, L. (1986). *Psychosocial aspects of AIDS: A component of family medicine education.* Workshop presented at the annual meeting of the Society of Teachers of Family Medicine, San Diego.

Herek, G. M., & Glunt, E. K. (1988). An epidemic of stigma: Public reactions to AIDS. *American Psychologist, 43,* 886-891.

Herz-Brown, F. (1988). The impact of death and serious illness on the family life cycle. In B. Carter & M. McGoldrick (Eds.), *The changing family life cycle: A framework for family therapy* (457-482). Boston, MA: Allyn & Bacon.

Hetherington, E., Stanley-Hagan, M. & Anderson, E. R. (1989). Marital transitions: A child's perspective. *American Psychologist, 44,* 303-312.

Heyward, W. L., & Curran, J. W. (1988). The epidemiology of AIDS in the U.S. *Scientific American, 259,* 82-90.

Hilgard, G. R., Newman, M. F. & Fisk, F. (1960). Strength of adult ego following childhood bereavement. *American Journal of Orthopsychiatry, 30,* 788-798.

Hill, R. (1972). The strengths of black families. NY: Emerson-Hall.

Hines, P. M. (1989). The family life cycle of poor black families. In B. Carter & M. McGoldrick (Eds.), *The changing family life cycle: A framework for family therapy* (515-544). Boston: Allyn and Bacon.

Hirsch, D. A., & Enlow, R. W. (1984). The effects of the acquired immune deficiency syndrome on gay life style and the gay individual. *Annals of the New York Academy of Sciences, 437,* 273-282.

Hoagland, J. (1984). Bereavement and personal constructs: Old theories and new concepts. *Death Education, 2,* 175-193.

Hodges. (1989) *Social Stratification.* Cambridge, MA: Schenkman Publishers.

Hodgkinson, P. E. (1982). Abnormal grief: The problem of therapy. *British Journal of Medical Psychology, 55,* 29-34.

Holmes, T. H., & Rahe, R. H. (1967). The social readjustment rating scale. *Journal of Psychosomatic Research, 11,* 213-218.

Hyman, R., & Woog, P. (1982). Stressful life events and illness onset: A review of critical variables. *Research in Nursing and Health, 5,* 155-163.

Jackson, E. (1979). Wisely managing our grief: A pastoral viewpoint. *Death Education, 3,* 143-155.

Jackson, M. (1980). The black experience with death: A brief analysis through black writings. In R. A. Kalish (Ed.), *Death and dying: Views from many cultures* (92-98). Farmingdale, NY: Bogwood Publishing Company.

Jacques, E. (1965). Death and the mid-life crisis. *International Journal of Psychoanalysis, 46,* 502-514.

Jayaratne, S., & Chess, W. A. (1984). Job satisfaction, burnout, and turnover: A national study. *Social Work, 29,* 418-455.

Jourard, S. M. (1971). *Disclosing man to himself.* Princeton, NJ: Van Nostrand Reinhold.

Jue, S. (1987). Identifying and meeting the needs of minority clients with AIDS. In C. Loukfield & M. Fimbres *Responding to AIDS: Psychosocial initiatives* (65-79). Washington, D.C.: National Association of Social Workers.

Kagay, M. (1991). Poll finds AIDS causes single people to alter behavior. *New York Times*, June 18, C3.

Kalish, R. A. (1985). The social content of death and dying. In R. H. Binstock & E. Shanas (Eds.), *Handbook of aging and the social sciences* (149-167). NY: Van Nostrand Reinhold.

Kalish, R. A., & Reynolds, D. K. (1981). *Death and ethnicity: A psychocultural study*. Farmingdale, NY: Baywood Publishing.

Kane, G. P. (1981). *Inner-city alcoholism: An ecological analysis and cross-cultural study*. NY: Human Sciences Press.

Kaplan, A. H., & Rothman, D. (1986). The dying psychotherapist. *American Journal of Psychiatry*, *5*, 561-572.

Karger, H. (1981). Burnout as alienation. *Social Service Review*, *55*, 271-283.

Kastenbaum, R. (1986). *Death, society, & human experience*, 3rd ed. Columbus, OH: Charles E. Merrill.

Katz, A. H., & Bender, E. I. (Eds.). (1976). Self-help in society--The motif of mutual aid. *The strength in us: Self-help groups in the modern world* (2-13). NY: New Viewpoints.

Kavanaugh, R. E. (1974). *Facing Death*. Baltimore, MD: Penguin Books.

Keefe, S. E., & Casas, J. M. (1980). Mexican Americans and mental health: A selected review and recommendations for mental health service delivery. *American Journal of Community Psychology*, *8*, 303-26.

Keith, R. (1981). Acute grief and survivor expectations. In O. S. Margolis, H. C. Reather, A. H. Kutscher, J. B. Powers, I. B. Seeland, R. DeBellis & D. J. Cherico (Eds.), *Acute grief: Counselling the bereaved* (206-207). NY: Columbia University Press.

Keller, A. S. (1988). Reflection on Hippocrates in a plague year. *Discover*, *8*, 26-27.

Kelly, J., & St. Lawrence, J. (1988). *The AIDS health crisis: Psychological and social intervention*. NY: Plenum Press.

Kelly, J. A., St. Lawrence, J. S., Smith, S. Jr., Hood, H. V. & Cook, D. J. (1987a). Stigmatization of AIDS patients by physicians. *American Journal of Public Health*, *77*, 789-791.

———. (1987b). Medical students' attitudes towards AIDS and homosexual patients. *Medical Education*, *67*, 549-560.

Kessler, R. C., & McLeod, J. D. (1985). Social support and mental health in community samples. In S. Cohen & L. Syme (Eds.). *Social support and health* (219-240). NY: Academic Press.

Kiapi, A. (1989). *AIDS, the law and human rights: A dilemma for the human race*. Unpublished paper delivered at Columbia University, New York Center for the Study of Human Rights.

Kielcolt-Glaser, J., & Glaser, R. (1987). Psychosocial moderators of immune functions. *Annals of Behavioral Medicine*, *9*, 16-20.

Kimmel, D. C. (1978). Adult development and aging: A gay perspective. *Journal of Social Issues*, *34*, 113-130.

King, M. B. (1989). Psychosocial Status of 192 out-patients with HIV infection and AIDS. *British Journal of Psychiatry*, *154*, 237-242.

Klein, S. J., & Fletcher, W. III (1986). Gay grief: An examination of its uniqueness brought to light by the AIDS crisis. *Journal of Psychosocial Oncology*, *4*, 15-25.

Knapp, R. (1986). *Beyond endurance when a child dies*, NY: Shocken.

Knott, E. (1989). Grief work with men. *Techniques and perspectives* (97-107).

Kohut, H. (1971). *The analysis of the self.* NY: International Universities Press.

Kolata, G. (1990). AIDS drugs is promising in study, but F.D.A. officials urge caution. *New York Times,* June 21, B5.

Kolata, G. (1991). 10 years of AIDS battle: Hopes for success. *New York Times,* June 3, A13.

Koop, C. E. (1987). Physician leadership in preventing AIDS. *Journal of the American Medical Association, 258,* 2111.

Kramer, L. (1990). A Manhattan Project for AIDS. *New York Times,* July 16, A15.

Krant, M. J., & Johnston, L. (1977–78). Family members' perception of communication in late stage cancer. *International Journal of Psychiatry in Medicine, 8,* 203-216.

Krener, P. (1987). Impact of the diagnosis of AIDS on hospital care of an infant. *Neonatology: Clinical Pediatrics, 26,* 30-34.

Krueger, D. W. (1983). Childhood parent loss: Developmental impact and adult psychopathology. *American Journal of Psychotherapy, 37,* 582-592.

Kübler-Ross, E. (1969). *On death and dying.* NY: Macmillan.

Lazarus, A. (1979). Unresolved grief. In A. Lazarus (Ed.), *Outpatient psychiatry: Diagnosis and treatment* (87-101). Baltimore, MD: Williams & Wilkins.

Lazarus, R., & Folkman, S. (1984). *Stress, appraisal and coping.* NY: The Free Press.

Ledger, W. (1987). AIDS and the obstetrician/gynecologist: Commentary. *Information on AIDS for the Practicing Physician, 2,* 5-6.

Lehrman, S. R. (1956). Reactions to untimely death. *Psychiatric Quarterly, 30,* 564-578.

Leming, M. R., & Dickinson, G. E. (1985). *Understanding dying, death, and bereavement.* NY: Rinehart and Winston.

Lerner, B. (1972). *Therapy in the ghetto: Political impotence and personal disintegration.* Baltimore, MD: Johns Hopkins University Press.

LeVine, E. S., & Padilla, A. M. (1980). Crossing cultures. *Pluralistic counseling for the Hispanic.* Monterey, CA: Brooks/Cole Publishing.

Levinson, D. J., Darrow, C. W., Klein, E. B., Levinson, M. H. & McKee, B. (1978). *The seasons of a man's life.* NY: Knopf.

Levy, L. H. (1979). Processes and activities in groups. In M. A. Lieberman & G. Bonds (Eds.), *Self-help groups for coping with crisis* (70-87). San Francisco: Jossey-Bass.

Lewis, J., & Looney, J. (1983). *The long struggle: Well functioning working class black families.* New York: Brenner/Mazel.

Lewis, L. (1984). The coming out process for lesbians: Integrating a stable identity. *Social Work, 4,* 464-469.

Lifton, R., & Olson, E. (1976). The human meaning of total disaster: The Buffalo Creek experience. *Psychiatry, 39,* 1-18.

Lindemann, E. (1944). The symptomatology and management of acute grief. *American Journal of Psychiatry, 101,* 141-148.

Lindemann, E., & Green, I. M. (1953). A study of grief: Emotional response to suicide. *Pastoral Psychology, 4,* 9.

Logan, S.M.L., Freeman, E. M. & McRoy, R. G. (1990). *Social work practice with black families: A culturally specific perspective.* NY: Longman Press.

Lomax, G. L., & Sandler, J. (1988). Psychotherapy and consultation with persons with AIDS. *Psychiatric Annals, 18,* 253-259.

Lopez, D., & Getzel, G. S. (1987). Strategies for volunteers caring for persons with AIDS. *Social Work: The Journal of Contemporary Social Work, 68,* 47-53.

Lovejoy, N. C. (1989). AIDS: Impact on the gay man's homosexual and heterosexual families. *Marriage and Family Review, 14,* 285-316.

Lum, D. (1986). *Social work with people of color: A process stage approach,* Monterey, CA: Brooks/Cole Publishing Company.

McGoldrick, M., & Gerson, R. (1985). *Genograms in family assessment,* NY: W. W. Norton.

McGoldrick, M. (1989). Ethnicity and the family life cycle. In B. Carter & M. McGoldrick (Eds.), *The changing family life cycle: A framework for family therapy* (70-90). Boston: MA: Allyn and Bacon.

McGoldrick, M., & Walsh, F. (1983). A systemic view of family history and loss. In M. Aronson (Ed.), *Group and family therapy* (375-385). NY: Brenner/Mazel.

Macklin, E. (Ed.). (1989). *AIDS and families.* NY: Haworth Press.

McNeely, R. L. (1988). "Five Morale-enhancing Innovations for Human Service Settings," *Social Casework, 69*(4), 204-213.

Mahler, M., Pine, F. & Bergman, A. (1975). *The psychological birth of the human infant.* NY: Basic Books.

Mann, J. (1989). Global AIDS in to the 1990's AIDS and human rights: Resource Material, *World Health Organization, 9.*

Mann, J., Chin, J., Peat, R. & Quinn, T. (1988). The international epidemiology of AIDS. *Scientific American, 259,* 82-89.

Margolis, O. S. et al. (Ed.). (1981). *Acute grief: Counseling the bereaved.* NY: Columbia University Press.

Martin, D. J. (1989). Human immunodeficiency virus infection and the gay community: Counseling and clinical issues. *Journal of Counseling and Development, 68,* 67-72.

Martin, J. L. (1988). Psychological consequences of AIDS-related bereavement among gay men. *Journal of Consulting and Clinical Psychology, 56,* 856-862.

Martin, J. L., Dean, L., Garcia, M. & Hall, W. (1989). The impact of AIDS on a gay community: Changes in sexual behavior, substance use, and mental health. *American Journal of Community Psychology, 17,* 269-293.

Marzuk, P. M., Tierney, H., Tardiff, K., Gross, E. M., Morgan, E. B., Hsu, A. & Mann, J. J. (1988). Increased risk of suicide in persons with AIDS. *Journal of the American Medical Association, 259,* 1333-1337.

Maslach, C. (1976). Burned-out. *Human behavior, 5,* 16-22.

———. (1981). The measurement of experienced burnout. *Journal of Occupational Behavior, 2,* 99-113.

Mass, L. (1987). *Medical facts about AIDS.* NY: Gay Men's Health Crisis.

Masterman, B. A., & Reams, R. (1988). Support groups for bereaved pre-school and school-age children. American Journal of Orthopsychiatry, *58,* 562-570.

Matthews, G. W., & Neslund, V. S. (1987). The initial impact of AIDS on public health law in the United States. *Journal of the American Medical Association, 2,* 344-352.

Merrill, J. M., Laux, L. & Thornby, J. I. (1989). Attitudes toward AIDS. *Hospital and Community Psychiatry, 40,* 857.

Meyers, M. F. (1981-82). Counseling the parents of young homosexual patients. *Journal of Homosexuality*, 7, 131-143.

Miller, M. (1985). Surveying the loss of a loved one: An inside look at grief counseling. In J. Frehling (Ed.). *Sourcebook on death and dying* (189-192). Chicago: Marquis.

Miller, P., & Ingram, J. (1976). Friends, confidants, and symptoms. *Social Psychiatry*, 11, 51-58.

Miller, S., & Dane, B. (1991). AIDS and social work: Curricula development in an epidemic. *Journal of Social Work*, 26, 177-186.

Miller, S. O. (1983). Practice in cross-cultural settings. In A. Rosenblatt & D. Waldfogel (Eds.), *Handbook of clinical social work* (490-517). San Francisco, CA: Jossey-Bass Publishing.

Miller, S. O. (1986). *Psychoeducation: A model for increasing social worker's help to families.* Paper presented at the clinical social work conference. San Francisco, CA.

Miranda, A. (1985). *The Chicago experience: An alternative perspective.* Notre Dame, IN: University of Notre Dame Press.

Miranda, M. R. (Ed.). (1976). *Psychotherapy with the Spanish speaking: Issues in research and service delivery.* Monograph no. 3. Los Angeles, CA: Spanish Speaking Mental Health Research Center.

Mizio, E., & Delaney, A. J. (1981). *Training for service delivery to minority clients.* NY: Family Service Association of America.

Modell, A. H. (1971). The origin of certain forms of preoedipal quilt and the implications for a psychoanalytic theory of affects. *International Journal of Psychoanalysis*, 52, 337-346.

Morin, S. F., Charles, K. A. & Malyon, A. K. (1984). The psychological impact of AIDS on gay men. *American Psychologist*, 39, 1288-1293.

Moss, M. S. (1984). *The last years of life*, Unpublished manuscript. Moss, M. S., & Moss, S. (1983-84). The impact of parental death on middle-aged children. *Omega*, 14, 65-75.

Murphy, J. (1988). Women and AIDS: Sexual ethics in an epidemic. In D. Corless & M. Leindenman (Eds.), *AIDS: Principles, practice and politics* (65-79). NY: Hemisphere Publishing Corporation.

Murphy, S. (1986). Stress, coping and mental health outcomes following a natural disaster: Bereaved family members and friends compared. *Death Studies, 10*, 411-429.

Murphy, Sister P., & Perry, K. (1988). Hidden grievers. *Death Studies, 12*, 451-462.

Nagy, M. (1948). The child's view of death. *Journal of Genetic Psychology, 73*, 3-27. Reprinted with some editorial changes in H. Feifel (1959), *The meaning of death.* NY: McGraw-Hill.

Navarro, M. (1991). *Women with AIDS virus: Hard choices on motherhood. New York Times,* 1 July.

Newmark, D. (1984). Review of a support group for patients with AIDS. *Topics in Clinical Nursing, 6*, 39-44.

Newmeyer, J. (1988). Why bleach? Development of a strategy to combat HIV contagion among San Francisco intravenous drug users in needle sharing among intravenous drug abusers: National and international perspective. In R. Battjes & R. Pickens (Eds.), *National Institute on Drug Abuse Research Monograph Series 80* (151-159). Rockville, MD: National Institute on Drug Abuse.

New York Times (1991). *Dying member of panel on AIDS wants her illness to lift stigma*, August 4, 1, 36.

Niederland, W. G. (1981). The survivor syndrome: Further observations and dimensions. *Journal of the American Psychoanalytic Association, 29*, 413-426.

Norton, D. (Ed.). (1978). *The dual perspective: Inclusion of ethnic minority in social work curriculum*, NY: Council on Social Work Education.

Oerlemans-Bunn, M. (1988). On being gay, single, and bereaved. *American Journal of Nursing, 88*, 471-476.

Olszewski, L. (1988). Survey of doctors find many reluctant to see AIDS patients. *San Francisco Chronicle*, July 7, A6.

Osborn, J. (1989). Public health and the politics of AIDS prevention. *Daedalus, Living with AIDS. Part II, Journal of the American Academy of Arts and Sciences*, 123-144.

Osterweis, M. (1985). Bereavement and the elderly. *Aging, 348*, 8-14.

Osterweis, M., Solomon, R. & Green, M. (Eds.). (1984). *Bereavement: Reactions, consequences, and care*. Washington, D.C.: National Academy Press.

Ostrow, D. G., & Gayle, T. C. (1986). Psychosocial and ethical issues of AIDS health care programs. *Q.R.B., 12*, 284-294.

Owen, G. R., Fulton, R. & Markusen, E. (1982-83). Death at a distance: A study of family survivors. *Omega, 13*, 191-225.

Palmer, E. L., Ramsey, R. B. & Feorino, P. F., et al (1984). Human t-cell leukemia virus in lymphocytes of two hemophiliacs with the acquired immunodeficiency syndrome. *Annals of Internal Medicine, 101*, 293-297.

Paradis, B. (1990). Seeking intimacy and integration: Gay men in the era of AIDS. *Smith College Studies in Social Work, 60*, 260-267.

Palumbo, J. (1981). Parent loss and childhood bereavement: Some theoretical considerations. *Clinical Social Work Journal, 9*, 3-33.

Parkes, C. M. (1972). *Bereavement: Studies of grief in adult life*. NY: International Universities Press.

———. (1975a). Determinants of outcome following bereavement. *Omega, 6*, 303-323.

———. (1980). Bereavement counseling: Does it work? *British Medical Journal, 281*, 3-6.

———. (1975b). *Unexpected and untimely bereavement: a statistical study of young Boston widows and widowers*. In B. Schoenberg, I. Gerber, A. Wiener et al. (Eds.), *Bereavement: Its psychosocial aspects*. NY: Columbia University Press.

Parkes, C. M. (1987-88). Research: Bereavement. *Omega, 18*, 365-377.

Parkes, C. M., & Weiss, R. S. (1972). Components of the reaction to loss of a limb, spouse or home. *Journal of Psychosomatic Research, 16*, 343-349.

———. (1981). Evaluation of a bereavement service. *Journal of Preventive Psychiatry, 1*, 179-188.

———. (1983). *Recovery from bereavement*. NY: Basic Books.

Patrick, P. (1984). Professional roles at risk for burnout. *Family and Community Health, 2*, 25-31.

Pearlin, L. I., Semple, S. & Turner, H. (1988). Stress of AIDS caregiving: A preliminary overview of the issues. *Death Studies, 12*, 501-517.

Peppers, L., & Knapp, R. (1980). *Motherhood and mourning*, NY: Praeger, Publishers.

Pilisuk, M., & Minkler, M. (1985). Supportive ties: A political economy perspective. *Health Education Quarterly, 12*, 93-106.

Pine, V. (1984). *Grief, dying and death: Clinical interventions for caregivers.* Champaign, IL: Research Press.

Pine, V., & Brauer, C. (1986). Parental Grief: A synthesis of theory, research and intervention. In T. Rando (Ed.), *Parental loss of a child* (59-96). Champaign, IL: Research Press.

Pines, A., & Kafry, D. (1978). Occupational tedium in the social services. *Social Work, 23*, 499-507.

Piot, P., Plummer, F., Mholu, F., Lamboray, J., Chin, J. & Marin, J. (1988). AIDS: An international perspective. *Science, 239*, 573-579.

Pleck, J. H., O'Donnell, L., O'Donnell, C. & Snarey, J. (1988). AIDS—Phobia, contact with AIDS, and AIDS-related job stress in hospital workers. *Journal of Homosexuality, 15*, 41-54.

Pollack, P., Egan, D., Vanderbergh, R. & Williams, V. (1975). Prevention in mental health; A controlled study. *American Journal of Psychiatry, 132*, 146-149.

Pyszczysnki, T. A. & Greenberg, J. (1987). Depression, self-focused attention, and self-regulatory perseverance. In C. R. Snyder & C. E. Ford (Eds.), *Coping with negative life events* (105-129). NY: Plenum Press.

Rabkin, J., & Struening, E. (1976). Life events, stress, and illness. *Science, 194*, 1013-1020.

Ramsey, R., & De Groot, W. (1984). A further look at bereavement: Abnormal grief and its therapy. *Psychiatry in Practice, 2*, 49-65.

Ramsey, R., & Noorbergen, R. (1981). *Living with loss, a dramatic new breakthrough in grief therapy.* NY: William Morrow & Company.

Rando, T. (1984). *Grief, dying and death: Clinical interventions for caregivers.* Champaign, IL: Research Press.

———. (1986). *Parental loss of a child.* Champaign, IL: Research Press.

Rando, T. A. (1985). Bereaved parents: Particular difficulties, unique factors, and treatment issues. *Social Work, 30*, 19-23.

Rando, T. A. (Ed.). (1986). *Loss and anticipatory grief.* Lexington, MA: Lexington Books.

Raphael, B. (1984). *The anatomy of bereavement.* London: Hutchinson, Basic Books.

Ratliff, N. (1988). Stress and burnout in the helping professions. *Social Casework, 69* 147-154.

Redmond, L. M. (1989). *Surviving when someone you know was murdered.* Clearwater, FL: Psychological Consultation & Education Services.

Reissman, F. (1976). *The inner-city child.* New York: Harper & Row.

Rodway, M., & Wright, M. (Eds.). (1988). *Decade of the plague.* NY: Harrington Park Press.

Rogers, D. E. (1988). Caring for the patient with AIDS. *Journal of the American Medical Association, 259*, 1368.

Ron, A., & Rogers, D. (1989). AIDS in the United States: Patient cure and politics. *Daedalus. Living with AIDS, Journal of American Academy of Arts and Sciences, 118*, 41-58.

Rosen, E. (1990). *Families facing death.* Lexington, MA: Lexington Press.

Rosenblatt, P. C., Walsh, R. P. & Jackson, D. A. (1976). *Grief and mourning in cross-cultural perspective.* NY: HRAF Press.

Rosenthal, A. M. (1990). *AIDS: The price of vendetta*. New York Times, March 18, Editorial.

Royse, D., & Birge, B. (1987). Homophobia and attitudes towards AIDS patients among medical, nursing, and paramedical students. *Psychology Reports, 61*, 867-870.

Rubenstein, H., & Bloch, M. H. (1982). *Things that matter: Influences on helping relationships*. NY: Macmillan.

Rudestam, K. E., & Agnelli, P. (1987). The effect of the content of suicide notes on grief reactions. *Journal of Clinical Psychology, 43*, 211-218.

Rudestam, K. E. (1977). Physical and psychological response to suicide in the family. *Journal of Consulting and Clinical Psychology, 45*, 167-170.

Ryan, C. C. (1988). The social and clinical challenges of AIDS. *Smith College Studies in Social Work, 59*, 3-20.

Sanders, C. (1984). Comparison of younger and older spouses in bereavement outcome. *Omega, 11*, 217-232.

———. (1982-83). Effects of sudden vs chronic illness death on bereavement outcome. *Omega, 13*, 227-266.

Sarason, I., Johnson, J. & Siegel, J. (1978). Assessing the impact of life changes: Development of the life experience survey. *Journal of Counseling and Clinical Psychology, 46*, 932-946.

Sattler, J. M. (1970). Racial experiment effects in experimentation, testing, interviewing and psychotherapy. *Psychological Bulletin, 73*, 137-160.

Savin, D. L. (1987). The expression of mourning in an eight-year-old girl. *Clinical Social Work Journal, 15*, 121-135.

Schaefer, C., Coyne, J. C. & Lazarus, R. S. (1982). The health-related functions of social support. *Journal of Behavioral Medicine, 4*, 381-406.

Schain, W. S. (1980). Patients' rights in decision making: The case of personalism versus paternalism in health care. *Cancer, 46*, 1035-1041.

Schell, D., & Loder-McGaugh, C. (1977). In S. Gerber (Ed.), *Children also grieve in perspective on bereavement* (66-76). NY: Arno Press.

Schlesinger, B. (1971). The widow and widower and remarriage: Selected findings. *Omega, 2*, 10-18.

Schneider, J. (1984). *Stress, loss, and grief*. Baltimore, MD: University Press.

Schoenberg, B., Carr, A., Kutscher, A. H., Peretz, D. & Goldberg, I. K. (1974). *Anticipatory grief*. NY: Columbia University Press.

Schoenberg, B., Carr, A., Peretz, D. & Kutscher, A. (1972). *Psychosocial aspects of terminal care*. NY: Columbia University Press.

Schowalter, J., Patterson, P., Tallmer, M., Kutscher, A., Gallo, S. & Peretz, D. (1983). *The child and death*, NY: Columbia University Press.

Schucter, R. S., Kirkorowicz, C., Zisook, S. & Risch, C. S. (1986). The dexamethasone suppression tests responses in the acutely bereaved. *American Journal of Psychiatry, 43*, 7.

Schultz, A. (1962). Multiple realities. In M. Natanson (Ed.), *Collected papers*, vol. 1, *The problem of social reality*, (207-259). the Hague: Nyhoff.

Shaffer, H., & Jones, S. (1989). *Quitting cocaine: The struggle against impulse*. Lexington, MA: Lexington Press.

Sheinberg, M. (1983). The family and chronic illness: A treatment diary. *Family Systems Medicine, 1*, 26-36.

Sherer, R. (1988). Physician use of the HIV antibody test: The need for consent, counselling, confidentiality, and caution. *Journal of the American Medical Association, 259,* 264-265.

Shilts, R. (1987). *And the band played on: Politics, people and the AIDS epidemic.* NY: St. Martin's Press.

Shneidman, E. S. (1981). Postvention: The care of the bereaved. *Suicide Life Threat Behavior, 11,* 349-359.

Siegal, R. L., & Hoefer, D. D. (1981). Bereavement counseling for gay individuals. *American Journal of Psychotherapy, 35,* 4.

Siegel, K. (1986). AIDS: The social dimension. *Psychiatric Annals, 16,* 165-172.

Silber, R. L., & Wortman, C. B. (1984). Coping with undesirable life events. In J. Garber & M. Seligman (Eds.), *Human helplessness: Theory and applications* (279-341). NY: Academic Press.

Silverman, P. (1981). *Helping women cope with grief.* Beverly Hills, CA: Sage Publications.

Silverman, P. R., & Copperland, A. (1975). On widowhood, mutual help and the elderly widow. *Journal of Geriatric Psychiatry, 8,* 9-27.

Simos, B. G. (1986). Loss and grief in family therapy. *Family Therapy Today, 1,* 1-7.

Sontag, S. (1989). *AIDS & its metaphors.* NY: Farrar, Straus & Giroux.

Spinetta, J. J., & Maloney, L. J. (1978). The child with cancer: Patterns of communication and denial. *Journal of Counseling and Clinical Psychology, 46,* 1540-1541.

Stehr-Green, J., Holman, R., Jason, J. & Evatt, B. (1988). Hemophilia-associated AIDS in the United States, 1981 to September, 1987. *American Journal of Public Health, 78,* 439-442.

Stephenson, J. A. (1985). *Death, grief and mourning: Individual and social realities.* NY: The Free Press.

Stevens, L. A., & Muskin, P. R. (1987). Technique for reversing the failure of empathy towards AIDS patients. *Journal of the American Academy of Psychoanalysis, 15,* 539-551.

Taylor, D. A. (1983-84). Views of death from suffers of early loss. *Omega, 14,* 77-82.

Terr, L. C. (1983). Chowchilla revisited: The effects of psychic trauma four years after a school-bus kidnapping. *American Journal of Psychiatry, 140,* 1543-1550.

———. (1984). Children at acute risk: Psychic trauma. In L. Grinspoon (Ed.), *Psychiatry update,* vol. 3. Washington, D.C.: American Psychiatric Press.

———. (1985). Children traumatized in small groups. In S. E. Eth & R. S. Pynoos (Eds.), *Traumatic stress disorder in children* (45-70). Washington, D.C.: American Psychiatric Press, Inc.

———. (1991). Childhood traumas: An outline and overview. *American Journal of Psychiatry, 14,* 10-20.

Thoits, P. A. (1983). Dimensions of life events that influence psychological distress: An evaluation and synthesis of the literature. In H. B. Kaplan (Ed., *Psychosocial Stress Trends in Theory and Research* (24-30). NY: Academic Press.

Thorson, J. (1985). Loss and adaptation: Circumstances, contingencies, and consequences. *Death Studies, 9,* 217-233.

Tiblier, K., Walker, G. & Rolland, J. S. (1989). Therapeutic issues when working with families of persons with AIDS. *Marriage and Family Review, 13*, 81-128.

——. (1987). Models of bereavement care. *Death Studies, 11*, 257-261.

Tooley, K. M. (1978). The remembrance of things past. *American Journal of Orthopsychiatry, 48*, 174.

Toupin, E. (1980). Counseling Asians: Psychotherapy in the context of racism and Asian-American history. *American Journal of Orthopsychiatry, 50*, 76-86.

Toynbee, A. (1976). The relation between life and death, living and dying. In E. S. Schneidiman (Ed.), *Death: Current perspectives* (324-332). Palo Alto, CA: Mayfield Publishing.

Treiber, F. A., Shaw, D. & Malcolm, R. (1987). Acquired immune deficiency syndrome: Psychological impact on health personnel. *Journal of Nervous and Mental Disease, 175*, 496-499.

Turner, C., Mailer, H., Moses, L. E. (Eds.). (1989). *AIDS: Sexual behavior and intravenous drug use.* Washington, D.C.: National Academy Press.

Turner, R. J. (1983). Direct, indirect, and moderating effects of social support on psychological distress and associated conditions. In H. B. Kaplan (Ed.), *Psychosocial stress: Trends in theory and research* (105-155). NY: Academic Press.

U.S. Department of Health and Human Services. (1986). Report of the secretary's task force on black and minority health. Washington, D.C.: Government Printing Office.

United Nation, Resolution. *World Health Administration, 41*, 24.

Vachon, M.L.S. (1976). Grief and bereavement following the death of a spouse. *Canadian Psychiatric Association Journal, 21*, 35-44.

Vachon, M.L.S., Sheldon, A. R., Lancee, W. J., Lyall, W.A.L., Rogers, J. & Freeman, S. J. J. (1980). A controlled study of self-help intervention for widow. *American Journal of Psychiatry, 137*, 1380-1384.

Valdiserri, R. O., Tama, G. & Ho, M. (1988). A survey of AIDS patients regarding their experiences with physicians. *Journal of Medical Education, 63*, 726-728.

——. (1990). The new horizon: Programmatic responses to the HIV epidemic. *Journal of Medicine, 88*, 219-220.

Van der Hart, O. (1983). *Rituals in psychotherapy: Transition and continuity.* NY: Irvington Press.

Videka-Sherman, L. (1982). Coping with the death of a child: A study over time. *American Journal of Orthopsychiatry, 52*, 688-698.

Volkan, V.D. (1972). The linking of objects of pathological mourners. *Archives of General Psychiatry, 27*, 215-221.

——. (1975). "Re-grief" therapy. In B. Schoenberg, I. Gerber, A. Wiener, A. H. Kutscher, D. Peretz & A. C. Carr (Eds.), *Bereavement: Its psychological aspects* (231-250). NY: Columbia University Press.

——. (1981). *Linking objects and linking phenomena: A study of the forms, symptoms, metapsychology, and therapy of complicated mourning.* NY: International Universities Press.

Walker, K. W. (1987). AIDS and family therapy: Parts I & II. *Family Therapy Today, 2*.

Walker, K. W., MacBride, A., & Vachon, M. L. (1977). Social support networks and the crisis of bereavement. *Social Science and Medicine, 11*, 35-41.

Wallack, J. J. (1989). AIDS anxiety among health care professionals. *Hospital and Community Psychiatry, 40*, 507-510.

Weinbach, R. W. (1989). Sudden death and secret survivors: Helping those who grieve alone. *Journal of Social Work, 34*, 57-61.

Weiner, R. S. (1988). Routine preoperative screening for HIV. *Journal of the American Medical Association, 260*, 179.

Weisman, A. D. (1973). Coping with untimely death. *Psychiatry, 36*, 366-378.

Weizman, S., & Kamm, P. (1985). *About mourning: Support and guidance for the bereaved.* NY: Human Sciences Press.

White, L. P. (1988). Educating physicians about AIDS—Let's do it ourselves. *California Physician, 1*, 6.

Wilcox, S. G., & Sutton, M. (1977). *Understanding death and dying: An interdisciplinary approach.* Port Washington, NY: Alfred Publishing.

Wills, T. A. (1987). Downward comparisons as a coping mechanism. In C. R. Synder & C. E. Ford (Eds.), *Coping with negative life events* (243-268). NY: Plenum Press.

Winnicott, D. (1971). *Playing and reality.* NY: Penguin Books.

Wolcott, D. L., Namir, S., Fawzy, F. I., Gottlieb, M. S. & Mitsuyasu, R. T. (1986). Illness concerns, attitudes towards homosexuality, and social support in gay men with AIDS. *General Hospital Psychiatry, 8*, 395-403.

Wolfenstein, M. (1966). How is mourning possible? *Psychoanalytic Study of the Child, 21*, 99-123. NY: International Universities Press.

Wong, H., Allen, H. A. & Moore, J. (1988). AIDS: Dynamics and rehabilitation concerns. *Journal of Applied Rehabilitation Counseling, 19*, 37-41.

Wood, G. J., & Philipson, A. (1987). AIDS, testing, and privacy: An analysis of case histories. *AIDS and Public Policy Journal, 2*, 21-25.

Worden, W. (1982). Grief counseling and grief therapy. NY: Springer.

Young, E. (1986). AIDS: Emerging moral questions. *Journal of American College Health, 34*, 240-242.

Zastrow, C., & Krist-Ashner, K. (1987). *Understanding human behavior and the social environment.* Chicago, IL: Nelson-Hall Publishers.

Zich, J., & Temoshok, L. (1987). Perceptions of social support in men with AIDS and ARC: Relationships with distress and hardiness. *Journal of Applied Social Psychology, 17*, 193-215.

Author Index

Subject Index

About the Authors

BARBARA O. DANE is Associate Professor in the School of Social Work at New York University.

SAMUEL O. MILLER is Associate Professor in the School of Social Work at Columbia University.